Aromatherapy *in the* Kitchen

Aromatherapy *in the* Kitchen

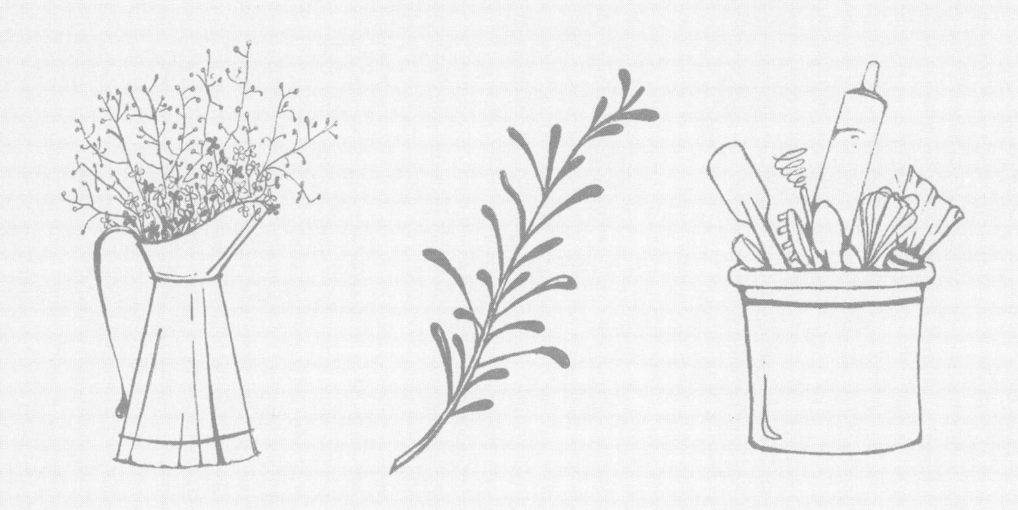

FRAGRANT FOODS FOR BODY, MIND AND SOUL

Melissa Dale & Emmanuelle Lipsky

Illustrations by KELLIE CANNING

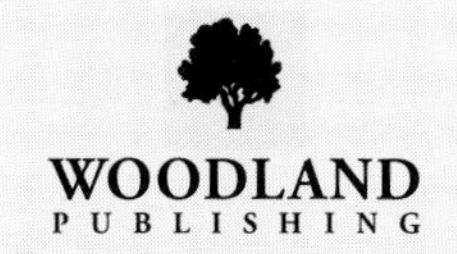

WOODLAND
PUBLISHING

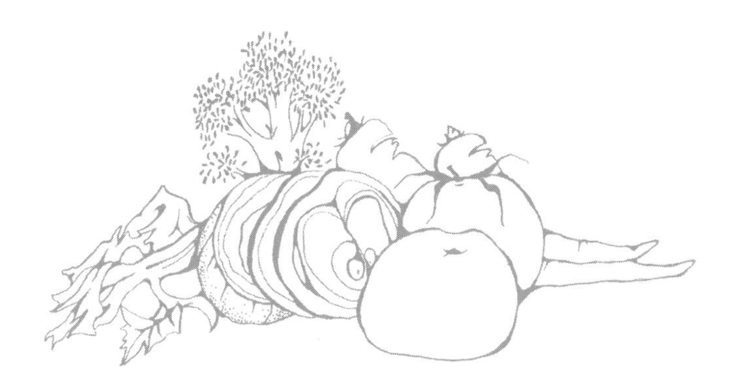

The CIP record for this book is available from the Library of Congress.

For ordering information, contact:
Woodland Publishing, P.O. Box 160, Pleasant Grove, Utah 84062
(800) 777-2665
info@woodlandpublishing.com

The information in this book is for educational purposes only and is not recommended as a means of diagnosing or treating an illness. All matters concerning physical and mental health should be supervised by a health practitioner knowledgeable in treating that particular condition. Neither the publisher nor author directly or indirectly dispenses medical advice, nor do they prescribe any remedies or assume any responsibility for those who choose to treat themselves.

ISBN 1-58054-348-0

Illustrations by Kellie Canning

Printed in the United States of America

Please visit our website:
www.woodlandpublishing.com

Contents

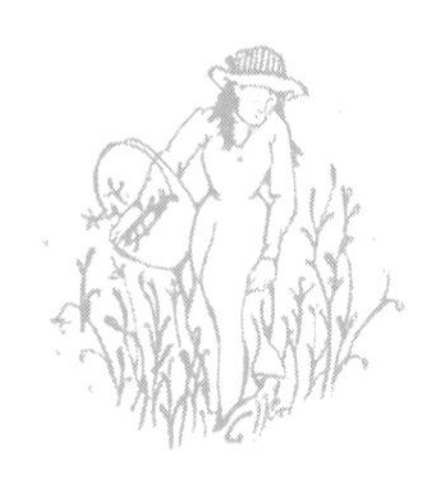

CHAPTER 1

AROMATHERAPY IN THE KITCHEN: Making Sense of Scents

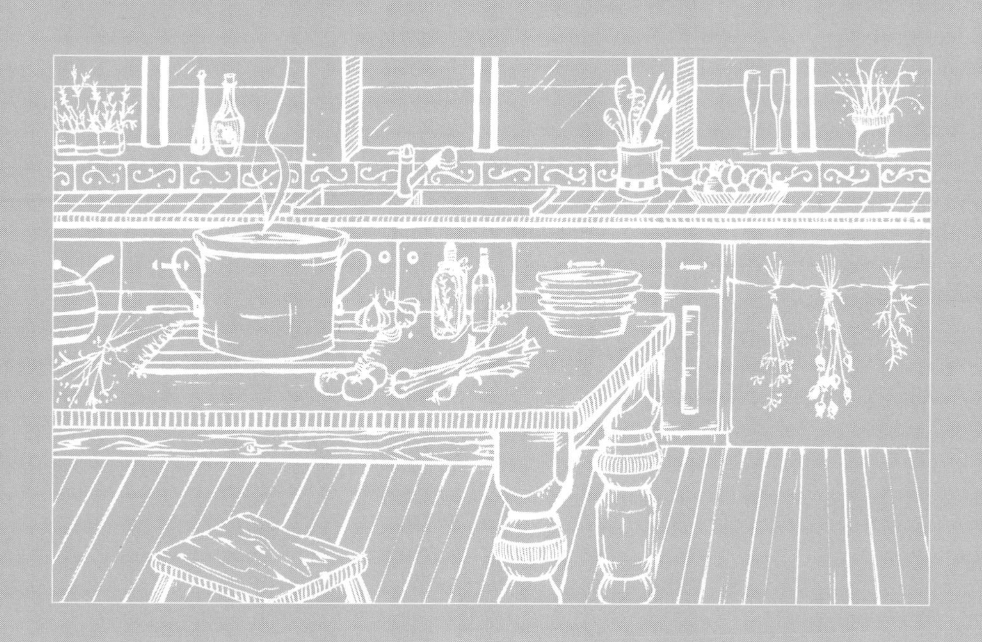

Introduction

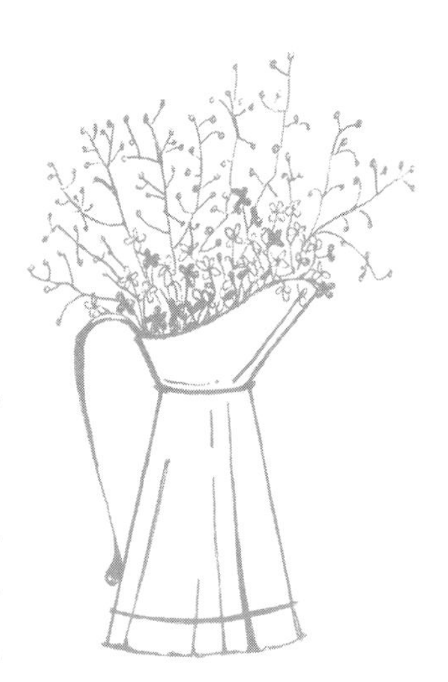

The benefits of aromatherapy are all around us—in flower and herb gardens; in air fresheners and scented candles; the perfumes, shampoos and other toiletries available to us from the cosmetics counter; and even in lemon-scented dish soaps and "pine fresh" cleaners. Aroma is used to enhance a massage and to scent an evening bath. It also helps us set a holiday mood or spark a memory of home. Chances are you have already taken advantage of at least some aspects of aromatherapy. Even a walk through a rose garden or brushing up against a rosemary bush can be therapeutic. In this book, we want to bring the benefits of aromatherapy into another realm—the kitchen!

Taste and aroma are intrinsically linked. Aromatics in food account for the vast majority of what we consider "taste." Without aroma, the flavor of foods would lack sophistication and uniqueness. We would be limited to the four basic tastes our tongue can detect—sweet, sour, salty and bitter. Anyone who has had a cold knows how bland food tastes without your sense of smell. Within any dish or beverage are a number of aromatics that contribute to its overall flavor. That's why wine tasters "swish" the wine in their mouths—to release these aromatics. They don't even need to swallow the wine to enjoy its complexity—they spit it into an urn. (We, however, prefer to go ahead and swallow!) We believe that since the aromas of herbs and flowers can positively affect the body and emotions in so many ways, why not use them to our full advantage?

What Is Aromatherapy?

Aromatherapy uses fragrant herbs, flowers and other aromatics to influence overall wellness through inhalation. By releasing the healing essences of flowers and other aromatic plants, we can positively affect our mood, emotions and physical health. Traditional aromatherapy uses essential oils, concentrated essences extracted from aromatic plants that contain the essential scent and life energy of the plant, but whole plants and their essences are also used.

Although the term "aromatherapy" is relatively new, scent therapy has been practiced for thousands of years. Though the practitioners in Mesopotamia and ancient Greece had not discovered the chemical and physiological ties between aroma and health, they practiced aromatherapy through an *a priori* knowledge that is well borne out through the discoveries of modern science. The benefits of aromatherapy are chronicled in ancient texts, which describe the wide variety of medicinal and household uses of herbs for balancing mind, body and soul. For instance, lavender, one of the most widely used essences, is not only a relaxing fragrance, but also an excellent remedy for headaches, stress and insomnia. Topically, it is used to treat acne and minor skin lacerations; aromatically, such as in sachets, hung bouquets, or potpourri, it repels moths and other bugs from a room, or in a drawer. In fact, the term "aromatherapy" was coined after French chemist René Maurice Gattefossé (1881–1950) discovered one of the therapeutic benefits of lavender. As the story goes, while working in his lab, Gattefossé suffered a burn. The only liquid nearby was lavender oil. He plunged his hand into the oil and was amazed at how quickly his burn healed. Afterward, he coined the term "aromatherapie."

There is also fascinating folklore about aromatic herbs. One story out of Greek mythology says that Hades, the god of the underworld, fell in love with a nymph by the name of Minthe. His jealous wife Persephone decided to put an end to his infatuation by turning poor Minthe into a plant. The grief-stricken Hades bestowed upon the plant an aroma that would forever be pleasing to all, and so Minthe became mint! We find it fascinating to integrate a love of cooking with the history, lore and aromatherapeutic benefits of herbs and flowers. We hope you share in our enthusiasms!

How Does Aromatherapy Work?

Recent research into the science of scent has uncovered many therapeutically active chemicals in essential oils and essences. The olfactory system is an intricate and complex mechanism. When we inhale a particular scent, it is picked up by two small patches of tissue on the top and sides of the nasal cavity, the epithelia. These patches are highly specialized, containing more than twenty million nerve endings just waiting to be stimulated by aromas as they waft by. The scent is converted into a nerve message that is immediately transmitted to the limbic system in the brain. The limbic system relays the perceived information from a particular aroma to the hypothalamus gland, which produces hormones. These hormones trigger both emotional and physiological responses.

Essential oils have proven effects on both the limbic system and the hypothalamus, especially in modifying mood, relieving anxiety and influencing sleep, but the therapeutic qualities of essential oils are far reaching. Just think about how the smell of a budding rose or perhaps the fragrance of a freshly cut lemon stimulates an emotional response. This is aromatherapy at work! Each oil has unique effects, and the inhaled influences of a scent may be different than its topical uses. For instance, you're probably familiar with the refreshing aroma of mint; topically, its essential oil can be used to treat bruises and as an antispasmodic agent.

A discussion of the complete physiology of aromas is beyond the scope of this book, and probably beyond the scope of our own knowledge, but simply put, there is a direct connection between the perception of aromas and the physical and emotional responses that they inspire. Still not convinced? Start using herbs, flowers and essential oils in your daily life (and cooking) and experience the magic as it has been practiced over the centuries. As this is primarily a cookbook, we encourage you to refer to the Resource Guide for a list of other good aromatherapy texts, as well as a list of suppliers of herbs and essential oils. Bring the benefits of aromatherapy into your daily life, not only through cooking, but in personal and household uses as well. The possibilities are endless!

Bringing Aromatherapy into the Kitchen

While cooking with herbs is nothing new, we wanted to bring the full sensory benefits of herbs, flowers and other essences into the kitchen in order to turn simple cooking into a complete aesthetic experience for the mind, body and spirit. Food preparation and feasting can and should involve all of our senses, so we decided to create a cuisine designed to influence mood using the principles of aromatherapy. Although traditional aromatherapy uses essential oils, we like to broaden this to include the practice of extracting essential oils directly into food through the preparation and cooking processes. The roots, leaves, stems, bark, flowers, seeds and fruit peels of whole aromatic plants contain the same essences used to make essential oils, and although less concentrated, they have the same therapeutic qualities.

Some people do use essential oils in the kitchen, but ingesting essential oils is still a controversial idea for many people, and it can be tricky. Culinary-grade, organic essential oils are often difficult to find; in fact, many labels do not specify the process by which the oils were extracted or if the oil is 100 percent organic. Furthermore, some oils should never be ingested, and others can only be used internally with caution. The concentrated flavor and aroma of essential oils make it far easier to over-flavor food as well. In order to get the flavor of an essence without the complication, most people use culinary extracts. Peppermint extract, for instance, consists of a small amount of peppermint oil diluted with water and alcohol.

We prefer using whole aromatic plants in our recipes because they provide the same benefits as oils but are safer and easier to use. We also enjoy the tactile sense of working with the plants, releasing their fresh fragrances, and having the visual presentation of the herb/flower in the finished dish. Essential oils can still be used in other ways to enhance the cooking experience, as we will discuss later. If you are interested in cooking with essential oils, refer to our Resource Guide for more information.

The key to using aromatherapy in your cooking is to let the effects of the ingredients work on you as you work with them. If you have planned a romantic evening, take advantage of the natural aphrodisiacs described in this book that will enhance your table—and your evening. If you need some energy, choose uplifting ingredients with invigorating scents to spark your spirit as you cook.

The recipes in this book are designed to be simple, elegant and pleasing to all of the senses, not just taste and scent. We have included more tips on creating an overall ambience for your dining experience by including other sensory details—like color, lighting and even temperature—to set the ideal mood. We invite you to join us in our celebration of the senses as we take the time to stop and smell (and eat!) the roses.

Infusions

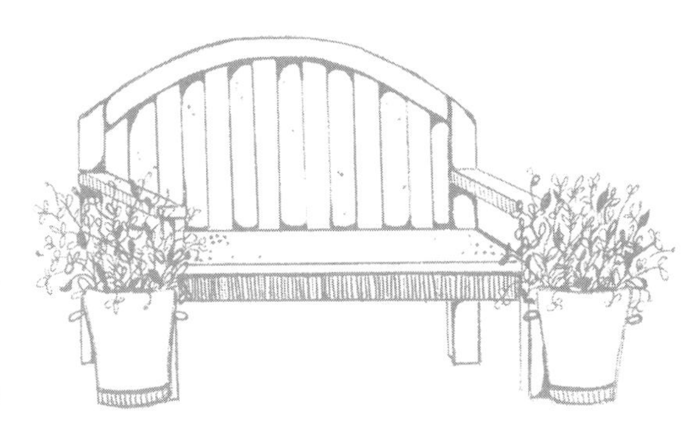

Infusions are a great way to get the most out of your herbs and flowers, and we use them in a quite a few of our recipes. An infusion is just a liquid like water or oil that is imbued with additional flavor and scent from aromatic plants. By steeping flowers and herbs in the liquid, the essences of the plants are extracted into the liquid. In this section, we will describe how to infuse oils and other carriers, such as crème fraîche or vinegar, which are often called for in our recipes. While pestos may technically be considered emulsions rather than infusions, we have included them here as they are another great way to combine fresh herbs with oils and are amazingly versatile. We have also included some easy and creative uses for your infusions.

Oils

Infused oils are very simple to make and are great to have on hand. Here's our advice: gather several small jars with tight-fitting lids (cleaned out mustard, caper or olive jars are perfect for this) to hold your oils. Do not use plastic

A WORD OF WARNING

Straining your oils is more than a recommendation. Although the idea of leaving your herbs and flavorings in the oil for visual appeal is tempting, it is not necessarily wise. Many herbs will begin to grow molds in oil, and raw garlic stored in oil can become toxic. The best way to strain your oils is to line your strainer with cheesecloth, which takes a little longer but will produce a clear oil. Save the presentation for vinegars, which are discussed later.

containers. A lazy afternoon is the perfect time to prepare a variety of infused oils, and it only takes a few hours.

Place a couple of large handfuls of your fresh or dried herb or flowers (less if you use dried plants) in a small saucepan. Select a vegetable oil with a neutral flavor, such as canola, grapeseed or corn. (Olive oils generally impart too much of their own characteristic flavor to use for this purpose.) Pour enough oil into the pan to cover the herbs or flowers. Heat over a very low heat for twenty to thirty minutes. The oil should have the distinct aroma and flavor of your herb or flower, and often carries a faint hue of the plants used, which is a visual plus. Let the oil cool, strain it into a jar, close tightly and store in a cool, dark place for up to three weeks. It's as easy as that!

We use infused oils in a number of our recipes, but there are infinite uses for these oils. Here are but a few:

- drizzle a little saffron oil over steamed asparagus
- toss fresh pasta with basil oil
- use an infused oil in your favorite vinaigrette recipe
- coat raw garlic cloves with oregano oil before roasting
- add some cracked pepper and fresh herbs to an infused oil and use for dipping bread
- mix jasmine oil with a little white wine vinegar and drizzle over artichokes
- use an infused oil for making your own flavored mayonnaise

Pestos

To some, pestos may seem caught in that awkward place between positively passé and retro chic. We happily ignore the naysayers and keep our food processors spinning out pestos on a regular basis. And though pasta with basil pesto will forever be a favorite, it by no means holds the exclusive rights for pesto use.

To make a basic pesto, place about two cups of fresh herbs in a food processor or blender. Add a few cloves of garlic, ¼ cup pine nuts and ¼ cup grated parmesan cheese, and pulse to blend. With the motor running, add a stream of olive oil until the mixture is smooth and well blended. There are, of course, unlimited variations of ingredient combinations.

PESTOS: FRESH IS BEST

Pestos can be made ahead and stored in the refrigerator with a protective layer of oil on top; however, they are so quick to make that we suggest preparing them the same day you plan to use them to get the freshest flavor and aroma from your herbs.

Pestos benefit from the character of the particular oil used. Try using walnut, peanut, avocado or hazelnut oils for a new twist. Pine nuts can be replaced with walnuts, filberts, pecans or whatever suits your fancy. Just remember to pair your choice of herbs, oils, nuts and other flavorings with the style of the food you're preparing—though it's pretty hard to go wrong!

Pasta is not the only pesto food. Here are some pesto possibilities:

- Stir some pesto into steamed rice for color, flavor and aroma
- Use pesto in place of butter for corn on the cob
- Swirl your favorite pesto into mashed potatoes
- Serve a dollop of pesto on grilled fish
- Pesto can quickly transform traditional popcorn into a special herbed treat
- Use pesto instead of tomato sauce on pizza

- Drizzle pesto over creamed soups for a gourmet flavor
- Spread pesto over savory cheesecakes or stratas

Vinegars

These days there are a myriad of infused vinegars available for purchase at specialty food stores and even at some supermarkets. They are so simple to prepare, however, why not just make your own? Infused vinegars placed in pretty bottles with colorful ribbons also make great gifts.

Simply buy a few pretty tall glass bottles (flea markets and kitschy antique stores are a great place to start) and cork stoppers with pouring spouts. Insert a few sprigs of your chosen herbs (and citrus peels if desired) and fill the bottles with white wine vinegar. The acidity of the vinegar keeps the herbs from molding, and these vinegars can be kept at room temperature for about two months.

In case the uses for infused vinegars aren't already popping into your head, here are a few more ideas:

- Create tasty marinades using infused vinegars as a base
- Use in reductions for beurre blanc or hollandaise
- Here's a stretch—use your favorite vinegar to make a flavorful vinaigrette for salads
- Splash a bit of herbed vinegar over steamed vegetables to give them extra flavor
- Try some with French fries instead of ketchup

- Replace your traditional vinegar with an infused one for pickling vegetables

Herb Butters

Classically called "compound butters," herb butters have been a staple in the culinary world for hundreds of years. In this health-conscious era, butter is almost akin to profanity, but we find that the use of both butter and profanities has an appropriate place in our lives when used in moderation! To make an herb butter, simply let a stick of butter soften at room temperature, work in your herb and maybe some shallots or crushed garlic, then roll it into a log on a piece of waxed paper. Seal it in a plastic bag and refrigerate until ready to use. Serve the butter sliced into disks. They look great and add an elegant touch to many dishes.

Below are some suggestions for using herb butters:

- Place a disk of herb butter on a piece of grilled chicken, fish or steak just before serving
- Add some zip to baked potatoes with a flavorful butter.
- Use decorative cutters to form the butter into pretty shapes for creative presentation
- Shave thin slices of herbed butter over steamed vegetables or fresh rolls
- Make a cinnamon and almond butter for pancakes or waffles.
- Use for making beurre blanc sauces

Creams

You may be thinking, as if butter wasn't bad enough, now we're talking cream? Yes we are, and again we evoke the age-old wisdom of moderation in all things. Cream has a unique and sensual taste and a palate feel that has no equal. Yogurt is a wonderful thing, and in some cases, it is extremely successful as a substitute for crème fraîche or sour cream, so if you must, you must, but understand that there will be change in character.

We have also experimented with evaporated low-fat milk (not condensed milk, there is a huge difference) as a cream substitute with varying results. Evaporated milk often requires additional thickening agents and has a taste and palate feel distinctly different from cream. It is, however, an option you can explore if fat content is a concern in your diet.

Infusing cream with herbs or flowers is accomplished using the same technique we used for oils. Floral creams make great bases for classic desserts such as crème brûlée or as an interesting alternative for making cream-based pasta sauces. Keep some infused whipped cream, creme fraîche or even mascarpone cheese in small plastic squirt bottles for a quick and artistic touch to a dish—savory or sweet.

Liqueurs are a classic and easy way to infuse heavier bodied creams. Simply stir in one or two tablespoons of your favorite liqueur into one-half cup of cream. Infusing these creams with herbs or flowers is a little trickier, but not much. Make a simple syrup by heating one-half cup water, one quarter cup sugar and a large handful of your flower or herb and allow to steep for twenty minutes. Then cool and strain. Use the syrup as you would liqueurs to infuse the creams. There are countless ways to use these creams, but here are a few ideas to get you started:

- Dollop some rose-infused crème fraîche over berries
- Add two tablespoons of basil cream to eggs before scrambling or making omelets
- Use rosemary infused cream for pasta sauces
- Garnish soups with a drop of herb-infused sour cream
- Use infused creams when making sweet or savory cheesecakes

Sugars

Infused sugars can be used in coffees, teas, crème brûlées, cookie doughs or anywhere else you would normally use regular white or raw sugar but want an added zip. Vanilla or cinnamon sticks can easily be inserted into a jar of sugar to impart their unique flavors. For herbs or floral infusions, first tie your herbs or flowers into a cheesecloth sachet, then bury the sachet into a bowl of sugar. The essences will release into the sugar over time. If you want to expedite the infusion, place your container in a window sill that gets some daily sun. Just make sure it's not hot enough to start melting the sugar! Below are a few ways to sweeten with herbs and flowers:

- Sweeten fresh lemonade with mint sugar
- Sprinkle fresh strawberries with rosemary sugar
- Dust fish filets with rosemary or lavender sugar when searing to create a great glaze
- Stir some vanilla or jasmine sugar into plain yogurt for an extra kick
- Use vanilla or lavender sugar in your favorite cake or cookie recipe

Infusion confusion?

Common sense and a little ingenuity are all you really need to start incorporating infusions into your daily culinary repertoire. Let your nose be your guide in creating fabulous perfumed infusions. If you have any doubts about what you are doing, browse through the recipes in this book and others to help you determine the appropriate use for particular herbs and flowers.

Helpful Hints

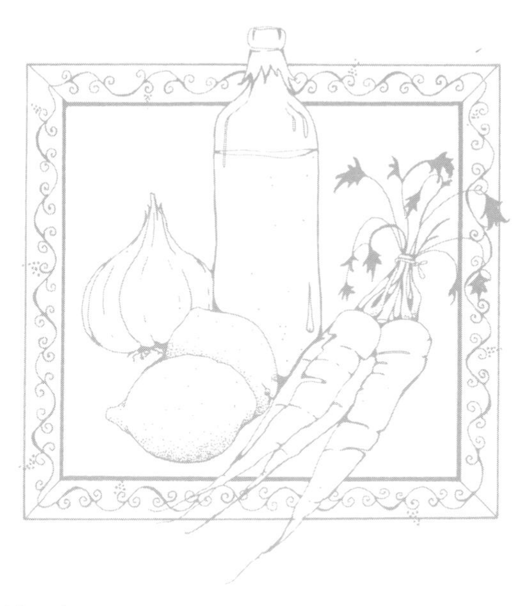

Ingredients

In order to get optimal results when cooking with herbs, it is always best to use fresh herbs. If fresh is not available, dried herbs may be substituted, but keep in mind that the quantity must be altered, as will be the results. Dried herbs impart a stronger taste (though not as fresh a taste) in dishes, so in general, use about one-third the measure that is called for in our recipes if you choose to use dried herbs instead of fresh.

Fresh flowers are harder to come by than herbs, however, so we generally call for dried flowers in our recipes unless otherwise stated. For suppliers of dried flowers and herbs, see our contact list in the Resource Guide or visit a local health food store. Of course, if you have a green thumb, by all means, cultivate your own culinary herb and flower garden!

Measurements

There may be some confusion about how measurements are written. There are measuring cups designed specifically for either liquid or dry ingredients. They are not necessarily interchangeable, so use the appropriate tool whenever possible—this is especially important in baking. Also, be aware of how a particular measure is worded. For example:

"1 cup basil, chopped" means measure the whole basil leaves first, then chop,
"1 cup chopped basil" means chop the basil first, then measure it,
"1 ½ c" means one and one-half cup, and
"1–2 c" means one to two cups.

Most people follow this basic convention, but it is worth reiterating just to be clear.

Tools

Knives. If you do not own at least one good quality knife, please trust us when we say that it is worth the investment! It's amazing how much more pleasurable your prep work is with the help of a good knife. If you can only have one knife, a six-inch chef knife is our recommendation. Henckel and Wustof are two highly reputable brands and can be acquired for a reasonable cost if you keep your eye out for sales. Check out the Resource Guide for a list of suggested retailers.

Food Processor. These days we make the assumption that practically every kitchen is equipped with a food processor.

If you are one of the exceptions, a sturdy blender can quite adequately perform most of the functions called for in this book.

Stand Mixer. Some of our recipes call for the use of a "stand mixer," by which we mean the classic KitchenAid style mixer, though there are other brands that work nicely. These mixers are not as common as food processors in home kitchens, so if you don't have one, don't worry! You can complete the tasks using a whisk or a hand-held mixer, although these methods take a little more time and effort.

And please don't forget that the two most important tools in the kitchen are your hands. Sure, you can turn on your 350-watt machine to work your dough, but until you feel that dough in your hands, you won't know if it's right. And without a doubt, there is no better salad tosser than your two (impeccably cleaned, of course) hands! Remember that cooking should involve all of the senses, and touch is an important one. Releasing the aromas of the foods you are working with through the touch of your hands is part of the pleasure.

Knife Cuts

There are classic culinary rules about the exact size of your chop versus your mince versus your dice. We don't keep rulers in our kitchens, and so we don't hold ourselves up to the strict rules of the culinary elite, though we admire them for doing so!

For general purposes, a vegetable chop is about one-half inch, a dice is about one-fourth inch and a mince is as small as you can cut it before getting tired! There is one classic cut, however, that we use regularly. It is called a "chiffonade" and is usually applied to basil or other large-leafed herbs. To make a chiffonade, layer four to five leaves of herbs on top of one another, roll into a tight cylinder, then cut across the roll to make julienned slices of the herb. This makes a great garnish for pasta, grilled fish and salads.

Mise en Place

This classic culinary term translates from the French to mean "put into place" and is one of the first things that is stressed in any worthy cooking class. It is a great practice to incorporate into your daily culinary routine. We have all watched cooking shows where the chef has a myriad of little bowls with perfectly minced garlic, chopped onion and whatever other ingredients are needed for their soon-to-be fabulous creation. Once they start cooking, everything they need is right there, ready to go. This is mise en place. Unfortunately, we home cooks don't have a staff to do such preparation, so we do it ourselves or corral a spouse or child to help. But once it's done, it makes the rest of the preparation a breeze! It also allows for some early cleanup of cutting boards and counter space so you aren't faced with a kitchen disaster after dinner. So, get yourself some little bowls, and do your mise en place—you'll be glad you did, we promise!

Creating the Mood

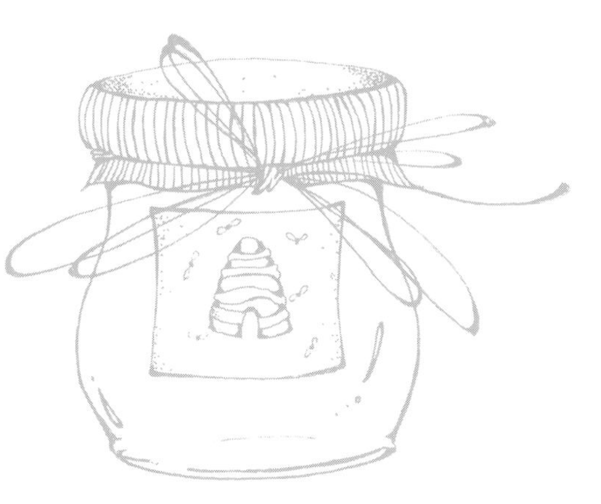

This book is designed to help you celebrate all of the senses, not just taste and scent. Creating an overall ambience for your dining experience means considering other sensory details to set the ideal mood. As you start to think about cooking with herbs and flowers to release the aromas that stimulate particular emotional responses, you might also consider what atmosphere best complements that desired mood. Whether it's a romantic dinner for two or a festive occasion with many guests, we have put together a few pointers.

First and foremost, beware of scented candles. Although they offer a pleasant fragrance, those fragrances are often synthetic. It is possible to find candles that use only essential oils, but be sure to read the fine print—some may use combinations of essential oils and synthetic scents. These candles may also clash with the scents of the food. Use unscented candles if you aren't sure. You've worked hard to promote natural scents through your cooking, so don't spoil it!

This does not mean that you should avoid candles altogether. Candlelight is an excellent visual way to set the mood. It not only enhances how we look, the soft light it creates also sets a relaxing or romantic mood. For maximum effect, don't limit your candle placement to the dining room. Place candles in adjoining rooms as well. Floating candles are another wonderful option—add a few fresh flower petals to the water in a clear glass bowl. You can color the water to correspond with your color scheme. Color is another essential aspect to mood that you can take advantage of. We will give you examples for using color later in this section.

Even though we don't advocate the use of scented candles, that doesn't mean you shouldn't enhance the aromas that will be wafting out of your kitchen. Use the fresh herb or flower you are cooking with to add visual and aromatic appeal to your dining area. Fresh herbs and flowers are pretty and can be placed around a room in all sorts of ways—be creative! Browse through flea markets and antique sales for decorative vases or small colored bottles to hold and display your aromatic plants.

Essential oils can also be used to perfume your room. Simply put a few drops of your chosen oil on a couple of pretty cloths and place them under a centerpiece, tuck them behind or under seat cushions or hang them in front of an open window to take advantage of a sultry breeze. You can also bring scents to the table by selecting your table napkins a day in advance and placing them in a shoebox or airtight bag with a few drops of essential oil. Just remember that essential oils are concentrated aromas, and a few drops go a long way.

Diffusers are another way to enhance the kitchen or dining atmosphere with your desired aromas. There are a number of varieties on the market. One of the simplest is a "ring diffuser" that you place on top of a light bulb. A few drops of essential oil are placed in the ring and the heat from the light bulb diffuses the scent. There are also some very handsome diffusers in which a small bowl is suspended over a votive candle. The essential oil (usually mixed with spring water) is placed in the bowl, and the candle's heat releases the aroma. There are also diffusers that are scented and plugged into electrical outlets.

Essential oils can also be added to humidifiers or made into fragrant room sprays using a spray bottle filled with warm water and a few drops of one or more essential oils. Room sprays are especially good for freshening carpets and curtains. For the more adventurous, consider adding one drop of cedarwood, pine or sandalwood essential oil to a plain log at least one hour before burning in the fireplace. (One scented log per fire is plenty.) Play around with some of these aromatic options prior to your evening of entertaining to find the balance that best suits you and the desired effect.

We have divided our recipe book into four categories: romance, refreshing/invigorating, relaxing and comfort foods. Here are our suggestions on how to create a complementary dining scheme for each.

Romance

A romantic dinner for two doesn't have to wait for a special occasion, and doesn't have to mean going to a spendy restaurant! Create your own romantic atmosphere at home with some fabulous food and some thoughtful preparation. You'll come out smelling like roses!

Color: Red immediately comes to mind when thinking of romance—red roses, red hearts and all things Valentine. Red is a great color to start with. It enlivens your passion, as it is an energetic color. Too much red, however, is, just too much red, so we like to blend in softer colors, such as pinks and taupe. Consider starting with a light pink tablecloth, and add some napkins in a darker shade of pink. Wrap the base of your wine bottle with one of your napkins for extra effect. You may also choose to place a bowl with floating heart-shaped red candles as a centerpiece. Some fresh rose petals strewn around the base of the bowl are a nice touch, or sprinkle some metallic red heart confetti around the table for a bit of whimsy. If you plan to use candlesticks instead, tie some sheer gold ribbon around the lower third of the candlesticks and let the ends of the ribbon drape in waves onto the table.

Dishware: Simple white plates look very elegant when placed on gold or silver charger plates. If you plan to serve your food at the table, select pretty serving dishes that complement your scheme. For a truly romantic setting, it is nice to have some classic stemware placed on the table—a water goblet, wine glass and champagne flute. And if you have special silverware that you never use, now is the time to use it!

If you're lucky enough to have a fireplace, by all means, take your dessert and champagne to enjoy in front of the fire. Our champagne-rose granita is a great way to finish your romantic dinner.

Invigorating

To create a lively and energetic atmosphere when entertaining, we suggest serving your food buffet style. The simple notion of having your guests mingle as they serve themselves promotes conversation and a sense of fun.

Color: We suggest draping the buffet table with a yellow tablecloth and accentuate it with a runner that has shades of orange, white and black (yes, black!) Black is an energizing color.

Scent: To help create an invigorating atmosphere, a combination of lemon and rosemary oils in your diffuser will enliven the mood. You can also use fresh citrus zests. Squeeze the zest to release the natural oils and place the zests decoratively around the buffet table.

Atmosphere: Decorate your table with a few bowls of

BUFFET BASICS

Plates should be at the start of the buffet, with silverware and napkins at the end. Serve drinks at a separate table or from the kitchen counter.

Have comfortable seating areas available to your guests. If your dining table can't accommodate the number of guests or if you just want to have some fun by creating unique seating areas, here are a couple of ideas. You could place some big pillows on the floor around your coffee table, and have people sit on the floor like they do in Morocco. Another area could be set up around a card table draped with a tapestry and adorned with a crystal ball and a deck of Tarot cards. We have found it fun to set up a side table with an array of unlabeled essential oils, with a small pad of paper in front of each of them. Throughout the evening your guests can smell the oils and write down their perceptions of the scents. It's a fun way to introduce people to aromatherapy and stimulate conversation. As always, be creative and let simplicity and fun be your guides!

pretty potpourri made up of dried fruits, leaves and berries. As for your lighting, we suggest it be bright, but not blinding. Consider replacing your regular lamp shades with Japanese lantern shades to bring color and diffused light into the room.

Relaxing

Stressed out? Know someone who is? We all get a little out of sorts from time to time, and wouldn't it be great if a friend or loved one took the time and effort to create a soothing and relaxing evening? Well, *be* that friend or loved one—even if it's for yourself! Here are some tips to soothe the aching soul.

Color: Linens in shades of blues, greens or purples help to promote a relaxing environment. If you have some scarves that fit your color scheme, drape them over lamps, over the backs of your chairs or simply let them flow together to make a beautiful centerpiece for your table.

Atmosphere: Put on some classical music, light a few candles, and start the de-stressing by offering tea towels that have been soaked in warm water infused with lavender essential oil. You can prepare the towels in advance and rewarm them briefly in a microwave oven. Bringing the lavender scent and the warmth from the towels to the hands and face will immediately promote a sense of relaxation. Follow this with some of our recipes from the relaxation chapter and finish the meal with a cup of chamomile tea and a couple of cardamom shortbread cookies. Short of a full-body massage, we can't think of a better way to de-stress.

Comfort Foods

As this category is subjective by nature, we leave it to you to decide what accoutrements best bring a comforting mood to your room and table. Just think back to your childhood and the aromas that greeted you when you walked in the front door—great food, a roaring fire and some mulled cider in the winter or a fired up grill and freshly squeezed lemonade in the summer. Whatever comfort is for you, keep it simple and from the heart and you can't go wrong!

Okay, we tried to be quiet, but we can't resist making a few suggestions . . .

Atmosphere: Go ahead and get a little retro. Bring out any old earthenware that you haven't used for a while and maybe a favorite heirloom tablecloth that is a bit too worn to use for company, but harbors warm memories for you. Place a low pillar candle as a centerpiece, and turn off the television. Put on some music you haven't listened to for years.

Don't fuss over serving your food—either bring your cooking pots or casseroles directly to the table or have everyone dish up in the kitchen and then convene at the table for an evening of great food and great conversation without fuss. It seems a bit of a lost tradition to have a family-style meal, even if that family is just you and a loved one. Still, that homey atmosphere is one we all love—and hey, it worked for Ward and June Cleaver!

CHAPTER 2

FUELING YOUR PASSIONS: Recipes that Inspire Romance

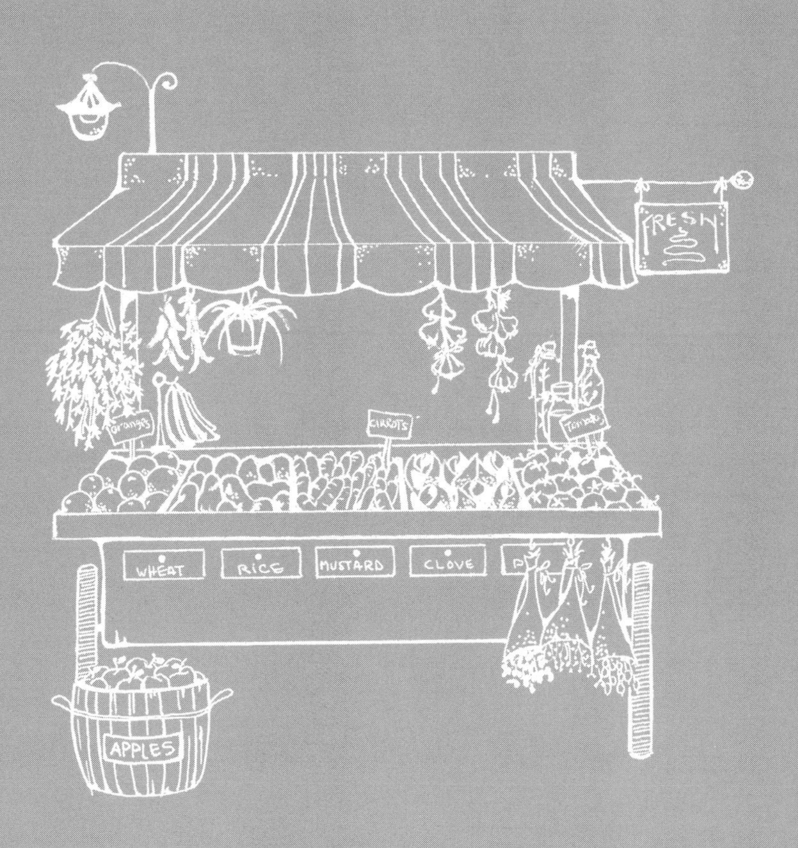

The Essence of Romance

The romantic "dinner for two" is a well-worn cliché, and for a good reason—it works! Creating a great intimate evening can be even better if you incorporate some of the wonderful and natural herbs and essences that are renowned aphrodisiacs. From the spicy energy of ginger to the tranquility of lavender, you'll find these recipes will enhance your dinner creations through the aromas they impart, the tastes they inspire, and the tactile nature of their handling. Breathe in as you cook, and be inspired—there's a lot of romance in the air!

Crab Gratin with Vanilla-Rose Oil

Serves 2 as a first course

This is so very simple to prepare, but oh, how it delivers! The aromas of rose and vanilla are a great start on your way to a romantic evening. We like this as an appetizer served with toast points and a glass of champagne. This recipe is for 2, but can easily be doubled or tripled if you're entertaining a crowd!

Vanilla-Rose Oil

½ cup canola oil
3 inch piece vanilla bean, split
1 teaspoon dried rose flowers

Combine all ingredients into a small saucepan over low heat and simmer for 15–20 minutes. Cool and strain.

Crab Gratin

1 shallot, minced
1 6-oz can crab meat, drained
4 tablespoons vanilla-rose oil
1 tablespoon half and half
2 tablespoons dried breadcrumbs

Heat 2 tablespoons of the vanilla-rose oil in a small skillet over medium-low heat. Add the shallot and cook until softened. Add the crab and 1 tablespoon more oil, and stir until heated and well coated. Transfer the crab to a small gratin dish (about 4 by 7 inches). Drizzle with the half and half. Sprinkle the bread crumbs evenly over the top, and finish with another drizzling of 1 tablespoon oil over the breadcrumbs. Place under a broiler until the crumbs are nicely browned.

Shrimp with Ginger Butter

Serves 2–4 as a first course

1 lb raw shrimp, shells on
1 stick (½ cup) butter
1 tablespoon minced ginger root
1 garlic clove, finely chopped
2 tablespoons chopped fresh parsley
salt and pepper

This very simple preparation pairs the ever-sultry shrimp with the sensuously spicy ginger to make a great start to a fabulous evening of romantic dining. Go ahead and get your hands a little messy with this fun and tantalizing dish! A loaf of crusty French bread makes a great accompaniment to soak up all of the delicious sauce!

Preheat oven to 400°F. Place shrimp in baking dish. Melt butter in a small saucepan. Add ginger and herbs and cook over medium heat for about 2 minutes. Pour over shrimp and bake in oven for 5 minutes. The shrimp should be pink and opaque. Remove the shrimp to a serving bowl, and drain the sauce into another bowl for dipping. Have ready a bowl for the shells, and a couple of small bowls with some water and lemon for cleansing your hands as you dive into this peel-and-eat appetizer!

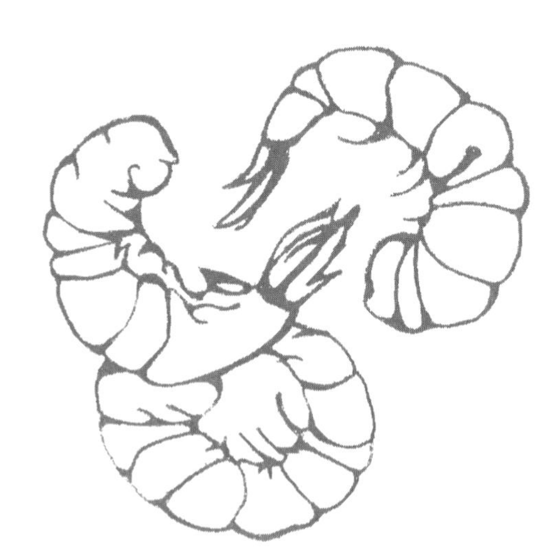

Basil Crêpes with Fresh Mozzarella and Oven-Dried Tomatoes

Serves 2 as a first course, with extra crêpes to freeze for later use!

WAIT, don't turn the page! Please don't let the idea of making crêpes intimidate you! They are really quite easy to master, and make for a great looking dish! (Of course you can pretend that you slaved over this dish—we won't tell!) The basil not only adds some great color to the crêpes, but also brings its aromatic qualities as well to create a truly romantic appetizer. Did you know that in old Italian lore, a woman would put a pot of basil on her balcony to indicate that she's ready to receive her suitor? Try putting a plate of these crêpes out instead, and wait for some awesome possibilities!

2 eggs
1 tablespoon olive oil
⅓ cup chopped fresh basil, plus 1 tablespoon for garnish
⅔ cup milk
½ cup flour

4 oz fresh mozzarella, sliced
2 plum tomatoes

For the Crêpes:
Have the eggs and milk at room temperature. In a food processor, blend together the eggs, oil, and basil until the basil is finely distributed. Stir in the milk. Place flour in a mixing bowl. Make a well in the center of the flour. Whisk in the wet ingredients until incorporated. (Do not overwhisk—some flour lumps are okay.) Transfer the mixture to a measuring cup for easier pouring.

Now for the fun part! Heat a 9-inch non-stick sauté pan over medium to medium-low heat. Lift the pan off the stove and pour some of the batter into the pan while rotating the pan to coat the bottom of the pan. Return the pan to the heat. When the edges start to curl up, flip the crêpe. The crêpe should be a nicely marbled light brown. Cook the crêpe for another 1–2 minutes. Slide crêpe out of the pan onto a sheet of waxed paper. The underside will have bright green flecks from the basil. (Don't panic if the first one doesn't come out perfectly—they never do!) Continue to make crêpes with the rest of the batter. The crêpes can be made ahead, stacked between sheets of waxed paper, and held until ready to use. (You can also freeze the crêpes in an airtight bag if you want to make them several days in advance to make your dinner-night preparation even easier!)

For the Oven-Dried Tomatoes:
Preheat oven to 375°F. Cut the tomatoes into 1/4 inch slices. Place on an oiled baking sheet (or if you want to cut down on dishes, make a throw-away sheet by doubling up a sheet of aluminum foil). Season with salt and pepper. Bake in the oven for about one hour, or until tomatoes are firm and dried, but not too charred.

For the Presentation:
Place a couple of slices of the fresh mozzarella onto one quarter of a crêpe, browned side up. Fold in half, and then in quarters to cover the cheese. Place on a baking sheet. Repeat with remaining crêpes (2 per person is more than adequate for appetizer portion). Heat in a 350°F oven until the cheese has melted, about 5–7 minutes. Place the crêpes on serving plates and garnish decoratively with the tomatoes and sprinkle the plate with some extra chopped basil. Now, that's amore!

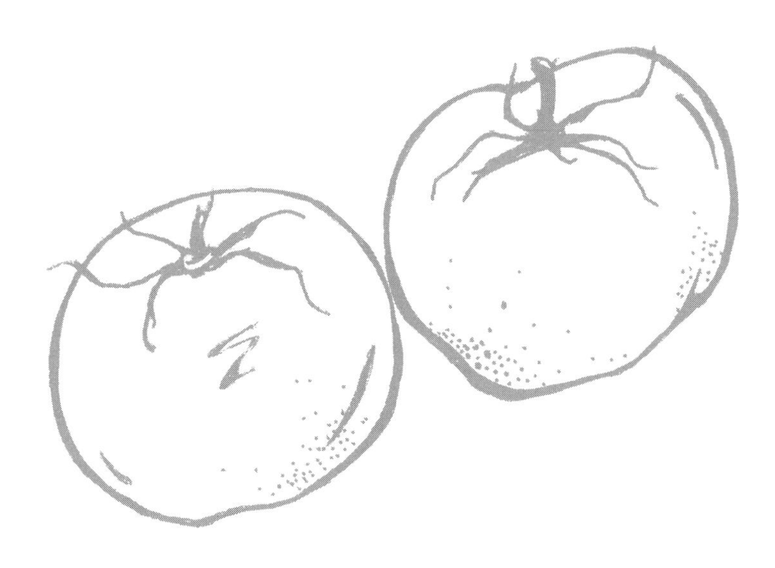

Gingered Scallop Timbales with Citrus Soy Glaze

Serves 2 as a first course

Ginger has long been considered a powerful aphrodisiac, and one whiff will tell you why! Its pungent and dizzying aroma plays well against the sweet and tart in the citrus soy glaze and the delicate nature of the scallops in this eye-catching (and delicious) appetizer!

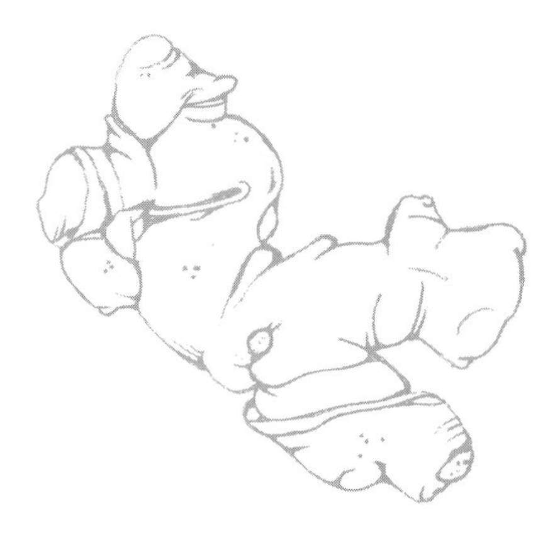

Citrus Soy Glaze

1 orange
1 lime
2 tablespoons sugar
1 tablespoon soy sauce

Juice the orange and lime, and strain into a saucepan. Add the sugar and soy sauce. Stir over medium heat until the sugar dissolves. Bring to a boil and reduce until thickened to a loose glaze, about 15 minutes. Remove from heat and cover until ready to use.

Gingered Scallop Timbales

2 tablespoons peanut oil
¾ cup couscous
¾ cup water
¼ lb bay scallops
1 tablespoon grated ginger root
1 tablespoon snipped chive
Freshly ground black pepper

In a small saucepan, bring the water to a boil. Add the couscous, cover and remove from heat. In a medium skillet, heat the peanut oil until hot, but not smoking. Add the scallops, ginger, and black pepper to taste. Stir until the scallops are just opaque, about 5 minutes. Stir in the couscous and chives and remove from heat. To make the timbales, press ¼ of the scallop mixture firmly into a 4-oz ramekin (or a small bowl). Invert the ramekin, whack it onto a serving plate, and slowly remove the ramekin to unmold the timbale. Repeat with remaining scallop mixture, placing 2 timbales on each plate. Drizzle the plates decoratively with the citrus soy glaze (transfer the glaze to a small plastic squirt bottle to make decorating a breeze!) Garnish with a little extra snipped chive.

Mesclun Salad with Jasmine-Seared Scallops

Serves 2 as a first course, or as a light lunch

8 shallots, cut into ¼-inch wedges
1 tablespoon jasmine oil
1 teaspoon sherry vinegar
⅛ teaspoon sugar

2 tablespoons sherry vinegar
6 tablespoons jasmine oil

5 oz mesclun (mixed baby lettuces)
1 pear, thinly sliced

½ lb bay scallops
½ red bell pepper, julienned
1 tablespoon jasmine oil

This is a beautiful and delicious salad that benefits from the aromatic qualities of jasmine oil. To make the jasmine oil, see the chapter on Infusions.

In a small bowl, coat the shallots with the jasmine oil, vinegar, sugar, and pepper to taste. Cook the shallots in a small skillet over medium heat until browned and caramelized, about 15 minutes. Remove to a small bowl. Place 2 pieces of shallot in a small food processor or blender. Add the remaining vinegar and the 6 tablespoons jasmine oil, and process until emulsified. Toss the mesclun and pear in a large bowl with just enough vinaigrette to coat. Divide onto serving plates and chill. In another bowl, mix the scallops and bell pepper with 1 tablespoon jasmine oil and pepper. Heat the skillet over high heat and add the scallops and bell peppers. Sauté until scallops are seared to a light brown and cooked just to opaque. Scatter the scallops, bell pepper, and shallots over the mesclun and serve immediately.

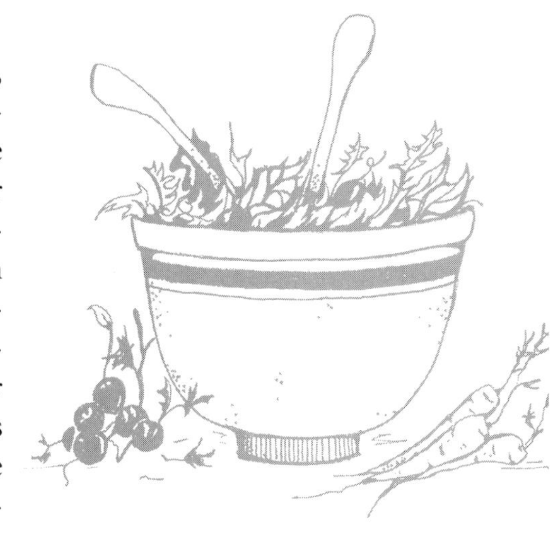

Lobster Salad with Basil Vinaigrette

Serves 2 as a main course, or 4 as a starter salad

There is a very old superstition which held that smelling basil would cause scorpions to nest in your brain! While the sultry combination of lobster with a creamy basil vinaigrette will surely have your head spinning, we're pretty sure that it's the flavors and aromas, and not scorpions, that are the culprits!

1 ½ lb lobster, cooked

2 tablespoons olive oil
1 lb baby potatoes (white, red, or a mix)
6 oz very thin green beans (haricots vert)

5 oz bag of mâche, or baby romaine lettuce

¼ cup fresh lemon juice
1 tablespoon Dijon mustard
1 egg yolk
1 ½ cups basil leaves
¾ cup olive oil
salt and pepper to taste
lemon wedges

Remove the claw and tail meat from the cooked lobster (you can buy the lobster cooked from your fish monger, or cook it yourself in boiling water for 8-10 minutes). Pull the meat apart into ½–1 inch pieces and set aside.

Preheat oven to 400°F.
Cut the potatoes into wedges, lengthwise. In a bowl, toss the potatoes with the oil, salt and freshly ground pepper until well coated. Transfer to a baking pan and roast in the oven, stirring occasionally, until golden brown and fork-tender. While the potatoes are cooking, trim the ends from the beans, coat them with the residual oil in the bowl, place on a separate small baking sheet (or a square

of aluminum foil) and roast until just crisp-tender, about 5 minutes. Remove the vegetables from the oven and allow to cool to room temperature.

In a blender, combine the lemon juice, mustard, egg yolk, and basil. Pulse to blend. With the motor running, stream in the oil and blend until smooth and emulsified. Season with salt and pepper. (Can be made a day ahead, stored tightly covered and refrigerated.)

In a large bowl, toss the lettuce with just enough vinaigrette to coat the leaves (use your hands—they are the best tool for this!) Add the potatoes, beans, and lobster with a touch more vinaigrette and gently toss to coat. Serve the salad in large shallow bowls with freshly cracked black pepper.

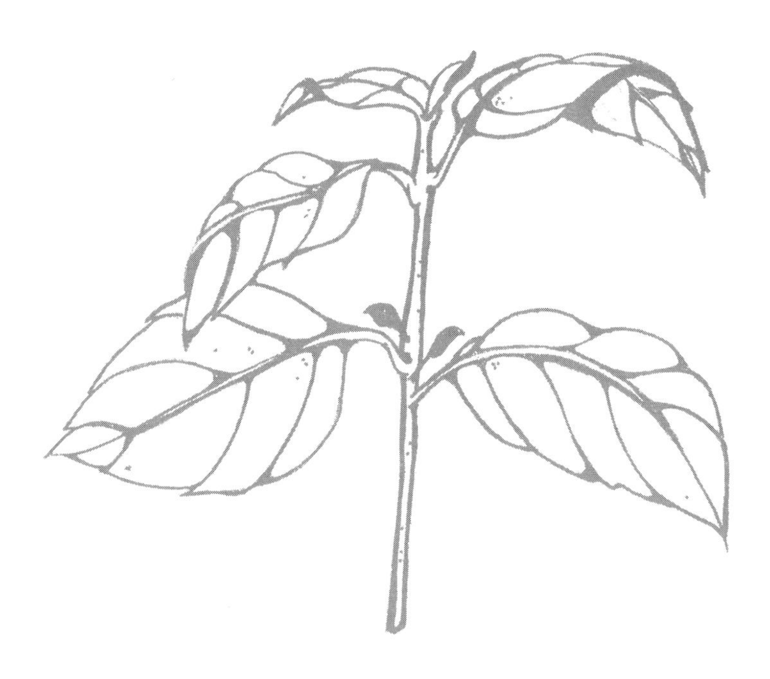

Lavender Roasted Chicken

Serves 4

Lavender is one of the most popular flowers used in aromatherapy. Its benefits are far-ranging, from providing antiseptic qualities through its essential oil to the calming effects of its heady aroma. It is equally as tantalizing in the kitchen, and is truly worth the effort to mail order some of the dried flowers for use in such elegant and sumptuous dishes as this simple roasted chicken. The smells wafting from the oven as it roasts are enough to drive you (and hopefully your loved one) wild!

3–4 lb chicken
1 lemon
⅓ cup dried lavender flowers
⅓ cup dry red wine
1 tablespoon flour
1 tablespoon water
salt and pepper

Rinse the chicken in cold water and pat dry. Place in roasting pan. Cut the lemon in half and squeeze its juice over the chicken. Put half of the lemon inside the cavity. Loosen the skin over the breasts and rub some of the lavender over the meat. Sprinkle the remaining lavender over the chicken and inside of the cavity. Roast at 375°F for 15 minutes per pound, until nicely browned. Remove chicken to a carving board and let rest for 10 minutes. Make a slurry of the flour and water. Place the roasting pan with the cooking juices on a stovetop burner and bring juices to a boil. Deglaze with the wine, and stir in the flour slurry. Reduce until thickened to sauce consistency. Carve the chicken, spoon on the sauce, and relish in the aromas and flavors!

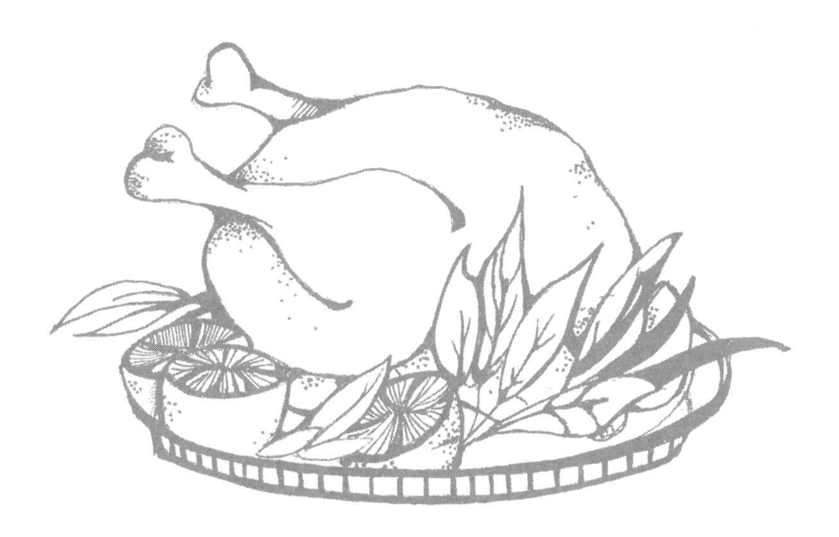

Truffled Mashed Potatoes

Serves 2, but can easily be doubled!

2 medium baking potatoes (about 2 lbs)
½ cup milk
1 tablespoon black truffle oil
salt and pepper

Truffles are not only for the very rich anymore! Thankfully, their much-lauded sensually earthy endowments are available in many markets in the form of truffle oil. White truffle oil is splendid drizzled over some risotto or a simple pasta, but for the richer flavor begged for in these potatoes, we prefer the more intense flavor of black truffle oil.

Cut potatoes into 1½ inch cubes. Place in medium saucepan and cover with cold water. Bring to a boil and cook until tender, about 20 minutes. Process into a bowl with a ricer, or use a masher. Add milk, truffle oil, and salt and pepper to taste and blend until smooth. (*Note:* do not use a blender or food processor to mash potatoes—they will turn into a gluey mess more suited for spackling than eating!)

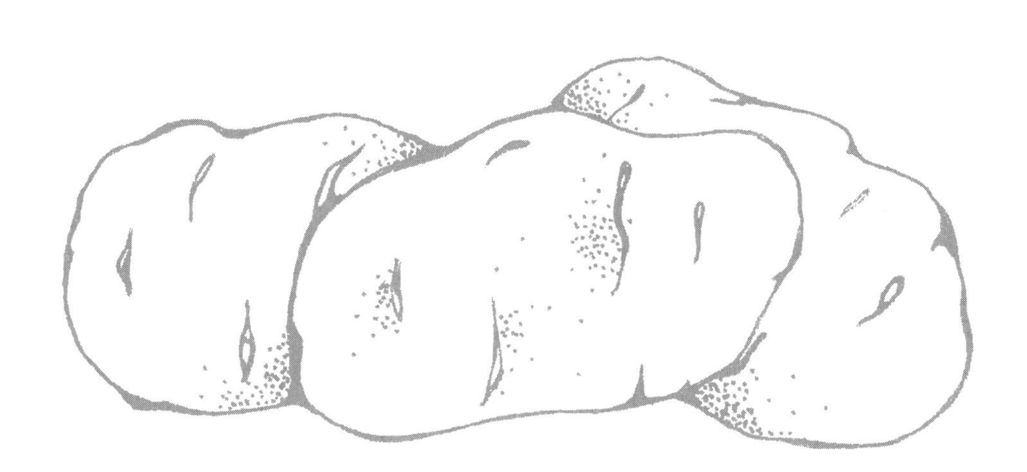

Mussels and Clams in Saffron-Bay Broth

Serves 2

Saffron. Need we say more? Saffron has an indescribable quality that has to be experienced to be truly appreciated. The color, the feel, the aroma, the taste—thank goodness someone figured out that it's well worth the Promethean effort to hand-harvest the stamen from crocus flowers! As an aphrodisiac we rate it among the top of the list!

6 large garlic cloves, minced
1 large shallot, minced
4 large bay leaves
½ teaspoon saffron threads
1 ½ cups dry white wine
1 tablespoon fresh lemon juice
1 lb mussels, cleaned
1 lb clams (butter or razor clams, preferred)

In a large pot, combine the garlic, shallot, bay leaves, saffron, wine, and lemon juice. Bring to a boil and let reduce for about 20 minutes. Add the mussels and clams, cover and cook just until the shells have opened, about 5 minutes (discard any mussels or clams that do no open!) Serve in bowls with a loaf of crusty French bread to soak up the broth.

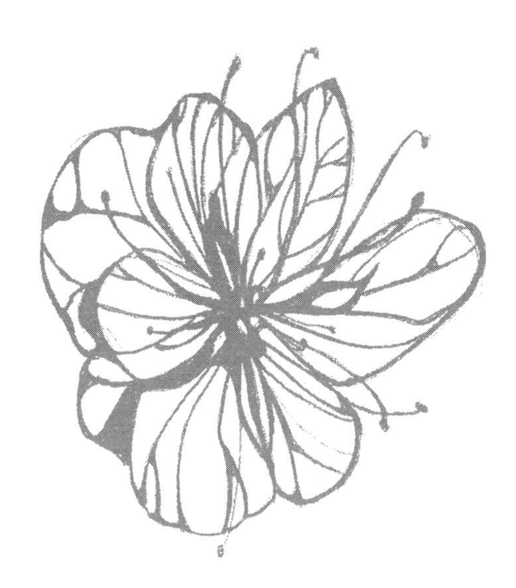

Jasmine-Seared Salmon with Pink Peppercorn Sauce

Serves 2

2 salmon filets, ½ lb each
2 tablespoons jasmine oil

1 shallot, minced
1 tablespoon pink peppercorns*
2 tablespoons raspberry vinegar
1 cup white wine, preferably Sauvignon Blanc
¼ cup cream
1 tablespoon butter
5–6 large fresh basil leaves, cut into chiffonade**

Jasmine is known as "Queen of the Night" because the luxurious scent of its flowers is most potent in the evening! In fact, the flowers are harvested at night to get the fullest body of aroma. Try making this jasmine-infused dinner one night and you too will be treated like royalty!

Coat the salmon with the jasmine oil and refrigerate for 20 minutes. In a small saucepan, combine the shallot, peppercorns, raspberry vinegar and wine. Bring to a boil and reduce to about 1/4 cup. While the liquid is reducing, heat a nonstick skillet over medium-high heat. Sear the salmon in the skillet, creating a golden brown surface on both sides, and cook until just opaque (about 5 minutes per side). Finish the sauce by adding the cream, returning to a boil for 5 minutes until thickened, and then swirling in the butter. Serve the salmon, drizzled with the sauce, and topped with the basil chiffonade.

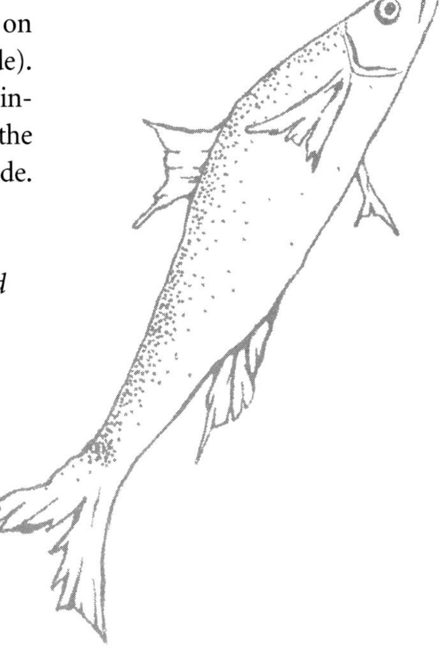

* *available at specialty food stores and some supermarkets*
** *to make chiffonade, stack basil leaves, roll tightly lengthwise and cut across the roll in 1/8 inch slices to form a julienne.*

Potato Galette with Truffle Oil

At the risk of mixing our moods, this galette goes extremely well alongside our Herbed Pork Chops with Port Reduction and a side of Green Beans with Oregano and Tomato—a great combo when you're not sure just what mood you're in!

1 large white potato (about 1 lb)
2 teaspoons olive oil
2 tablespoons black truffle oil
salt and pepper to taste

Thinly slice the potato and put into a bowl of ice water. Drain the potato slices, pat dry, and return to the bowl. Drizzle with the olive oil, 1 tablespoon of the truffle oil, and salt and pepper to taste, and toss until well coated. Arrange the potatoes in rounds in a 9-inch nonstick skillet. Cover with foil and weight the pan with a cast iron skillet, a brick, or whatever heavy implement you have on hand that will fit over the potatoes! Let the potatoes sit under the weights for 20 minutes. Place the pan on a burner over medium-high heat. Let cook, still weighted, for 10 minutes, or until the underside is browned and crispy. Remove the weight and foil, drizzle with the remaining 1 tablespoon truffle oil, and reseason with salt and pepper. Place a large plate over the pan, and invert the potatoes onto the plate. Slide the galette back into the pan and continue cooking, uncovered, until the bottom side is browned and the potatoes are cooked through. Cut into wedges and serve.

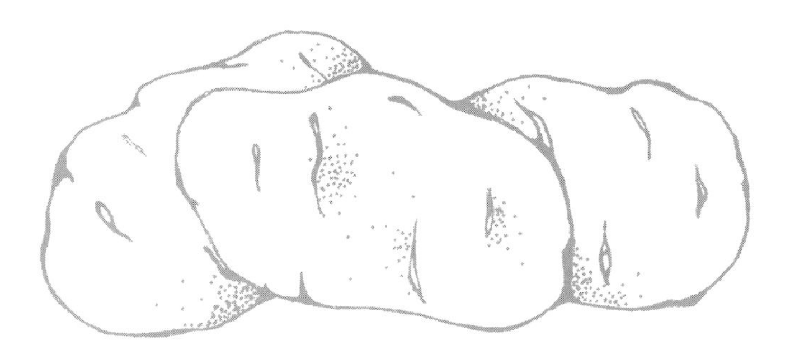

Lavender Chicken with Fresh Figs

Serves 4–6

3 tablespoons olive oil
6 boneless chicken breast halves
½ cup white wine
8–10 fresh figs, cut into quarters
4 garlic cloves, quartered
3 tablespoons dried lavender flowers, minced
1 tablespoon lavender leaves, minced
1 cup chicken broth
3 tablespoons honey
salt and pepper

In ancient times, lavender was commonly given as a gift of affection. You can make up some bouquets of fresh lavender to have ready for your dinner companions as gifts to take home—as well as preparing the gift of food! Here's another great pairing of lavender and chicken, this time with the lovely addition of fresh figs.

In a large saucepan, heat the oil over medium heat. Season the chicken with salt and pepper, and brown on both sides. Add the wine and figs, increase the heat to high, and bring to a boil. Return to medium heat, add the lavender flowers and leaves, garlic and honey. Cover and cook for 10 minutes. Remove the lid and cook for an additional 10 minutes, or until the chicken is just cooked through. Serve over rice or couscous garnished with a few lavender flowers.

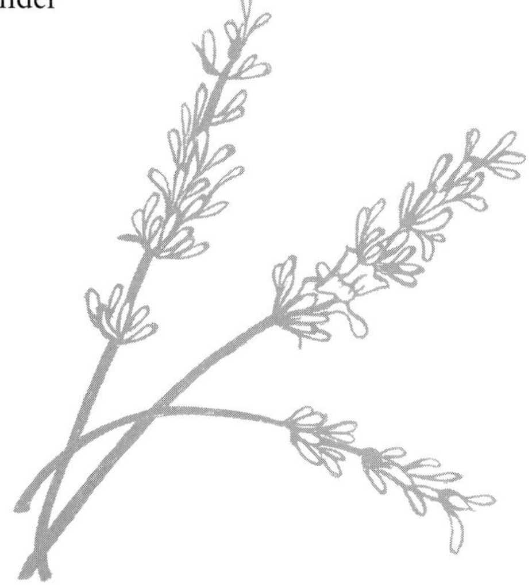

Morel Crusted Game Hens

Serves 2–4

Morel mushrooms are highly prized for their depth of character—robust, sultry, and intoxicating in both aroma and flavor. Unfortunately, they are also highly priced, but not to worry—in this preparation we have extracted a lot of bang for very little bucks! Black truffle oil adds yet another layer of deep mushroom tones to enhance your dining experience to a state of romantic euphoria!

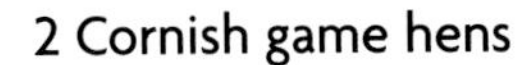

2 Cornish game hens
¼ oz dried morel mushrooms (about 4 medium mushrooms)
¼ teaspoon cumin
¼ teaspoon ground sage
¼ teaspoon freshly ground black pepper
⅛ teaspoon salt
¼ cup black truffle oil
¼ cup dry white wine
2 teaspoons cornstarch
1 tablespoon cold water

Grind the morel mushrooms in a spice blender or coffee grinder until they are finely ground. Add the cumin, sage, pepper, and salt and process until well blended. Set aside.

Preheat oven to 500°F. Brush hens all over with truffle oil. Place the hens breast-side down on a broiler pan fitted over a drip pan. Place in the oven and cook until the skin starts to sear, about 5 minutes. Turn breast-side up and return to oven until breast side starts to brown, another 5 minutes. Remove from oven and reduce heat to 425°F.

Pour any juices from the drip pan into a small saucepan. Re-position the hens breast-side down, brush with truffle oil, and sprinkle with half of the mushroom mixture. Bake for 12 minutes. Remove from oven and turn breast-side up. Brush the breast side with truffle oil, sprinkle with the remaining mushroom mix, and return to the oven for another 12 minutes, or until the breasts are browned and the juices run clear. Remove from the oven, place the hens on a cutting board and deglaze the drip pan with the wine. Add the deglazing liquid to the saucepan with the juices, and bring to a boil. Make a slurry with the cornstarch and the cold water, and add to the sauce to thicken. Cut each hen in half and serve with the sauce.

Shrimp and Sausage Paella

Serves 4

2 links sausage (use your favorite), cut into ½ inch slices
¼ cup olive oil
1 onion, chopped
4 garlic cloves, minced
½ cup mushrooms, sliced
2 ½ cups Arborio rice
¼–½ teaspoon saffron threads
5 cups water (or vegetable broth)
¾ cup red bell pepper, diced
¾ cup frozen peas, thawed
¾ cup frozen corn, thawed
12 large raw shrimp, peeled and deveined
2 tablespoons chopped parsley
lemon wedges, for garnish

Paella is a fabulous one-dish meal that is as appealing to the eye as it is to the palate! Saffron imparts a great yellow color to the rice as well as its intensely sensual aroma and flavor!

In a 2½ quart pot or paella pan, cook the sausage over medium high heat until browned and cooked through. Remove to a plate lined with a paper towel to drain. Wipe any excess grease from the pan, return to heat and pour in the olive oil. Sauté the onion and garlic in the oil until translucent. Add the mushrooms and rice, and stir until well coated. Crush the saffron threads over the rice and cook, stirring, until the rice is translucent. Add the water, bring to a boil, then cover and reduce the heat to low. Cook for about 25 minutes, or until the liquid is nearly all absorbed and the rice is still a bit hard to the bite. Stir in the bell pepper, peas, and corn, cover and continue cooking for about 5 minutes. Press the shrimp into the rice, cover, and cook until the shrimp are just opaque and the rice is tender to the bite, about another 5 minutes. Sprinkle with the parsley. Bring the cooking pot to the table and serve the paella in large shallow bowls with the lemon wedges.

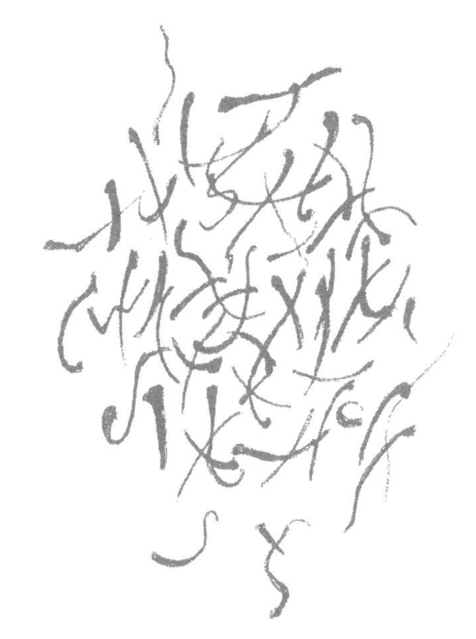

Gnocchi with Chicken and Portobellos

Serves 2

One of the many attributes of basil is that of being an herb of love (we like that one!) We find this to be a cozy dish for two, served with some warm crusty bread and a nice Cabernet.

2 boneless skinless chicken breast halves
2 garlic cloves, crushed
1 teaspoon lemon pepper
¼ cup basil oil*

4 pearl or roma tomatoes, quartered
¼ lb asparagus tips
¼ cup chopped basil
1 tablespoon sherry vinegar
1 tablespoon basil oil

2 portobello mushrooms (about 6 oz total)

1 lb gnocchi**

shaved parmesan

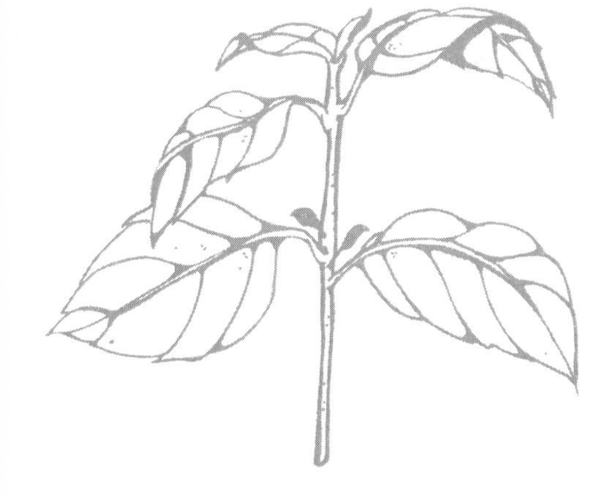

In a shallow dish, rub the chicken with the crushed garlic, lemon pepper, and basil oil, and let marinate chilled for 20 minutes.
Toss the tomatoes, asparagus, and basil with the sherry vinegar and basil oil in a glass bowl and set aside covered with plastic wrap at room temperature.

Bring a large pot of water to a gentle boil and cook the gnocchi until they float. Drain and drizzle with a little basil oil to prevent sticking. While the gnocchi are cooking, heat a skillet over medium-high heat. Place the chicken in the pan, sear on both sides, then reduce heat to medium. Cut the mushrooms into half-inch slices and brush with any chicken marinade that is left in the dish. Cook the mushrooms alongside the chicken until they are soft and browned, and until the chicken is cooked through. Remove the chicken and mushrooms to a cutting board. Increase the heat to high and sauté the tomato and asparagus mixture for 5 minutes, or until the asparagus is just tender to the bite. Toss the tomato mixture with the gnocchi and divide into large shallow bowls. Slice the chicken breasts into half-inch slices, fan the chicken and the mushrooms over the gnocchi, and garnish with shaved parmesan.

**basil oil is available in specialty food stores, or better yet, make your own—see our chapter on infusions!*
***gnocchi can be found frozen or vacuum-packed in specialty food stores and some supermarkets*

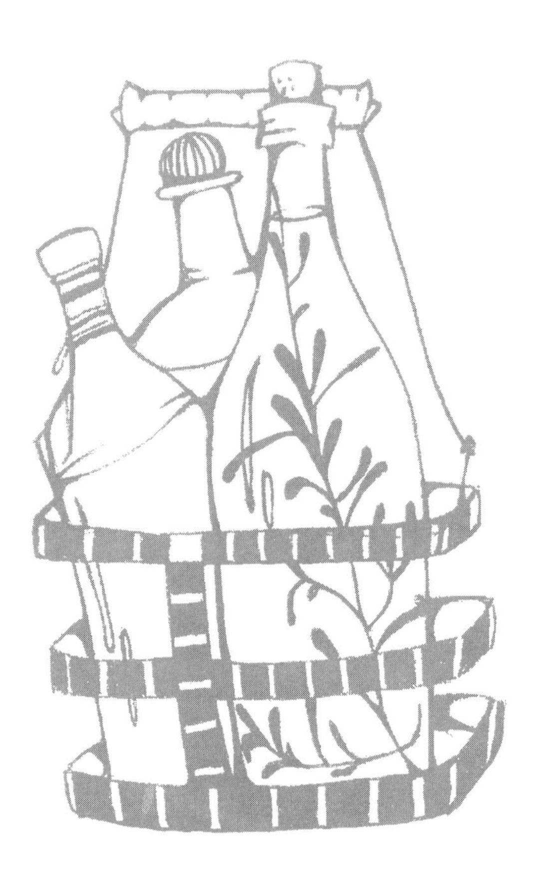

Shrimp Pesto Pizza

Serves 4

Okay, we know—using a prepared pizza dough is cheating, but when time is of the essence, it sure comes in handy! Use freshly made pesto to really bring out the aromas and flavor of the basil. This pizza comes out looking as great as it tastes!

1 prepared pizza shell
6 jumbo shrimp, halved lengthwise
3 garlic cloves, sliced
1 cup sliced mushrooms
¼ cup sliced sundried tomatoes (packed in oil, drained)
¼ cup sliced roasted red bell peppers
¼ cup homemade basil pesto
½ cup mozzarella cheese
¼ cup fresh spinach leaves
2 tablespoons pine nuts

Toss the shrimp with 1 tablespoon pesto and set aside. Drain about 2 teaspoons oil from the sundried tomatoes into a small skillet. Heat over medium-high heat and sauté the garlic, mushrooms, sundried tomatoes, and roasted peppers for 5 minutes. Remove from heat.

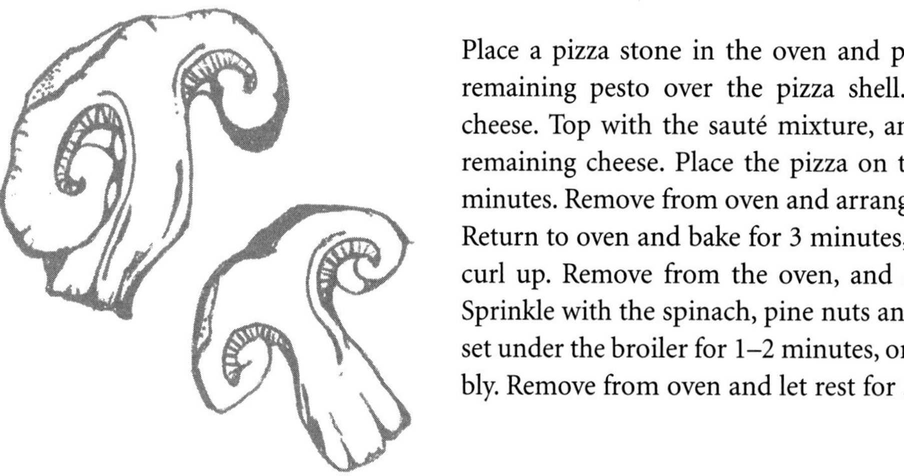

Place a pizza stone in the oven and preheat to 425°F. Spread the remaining pesto over the pizza shell. Sprinkle with half of the cheese. Top with the sauté mixture, and sprinkle with half of the remaining cheese. Place the pizza on the stone and bake for 8-10 minutes. Remove from oven and arrange the shrimp over the pizza. Return to oven and bake for 3 minutes, or until the shrimp start to curl up. Remove from the oven, and set the thermostat to broil. Sprinkle with the spinach, pine nuts and the remaining cheese, and set under the broiler for 1–2 minutes, or until the cheese is just bubbly. Remove from oven and let rest for 3–5 minutes before slicing.

Mango-Lavender Sorbet

1 cup spring water
⅓ cup sugar
1 tablespoon dried lavender
4 cups cubed mango

This sorbet is a pretty and light way to end a sumptuous romantic dinner! Try serving it in a single dessert dish with two long-handled spoons, perhaps garnished with some perfect red raspberries and a sprig of fresh lavender.

Place an 8-inch square metal pan in the freezer.
In a small saucepan, heat the water, sugar and lavender until just boiling. Remove from heat and let cool to room temperature. Strain into a bowl and refrigerate until cooled. Puree the mango in a food processor until smooth. Add the syrup and blend. Pour into the cold pan and place in freezer. After one hour, stir vigorously with a fork. Return to freezer and chill until firmly set, about 3 hours. (Alternately, the sorbet can be processed in an ice cream machine).

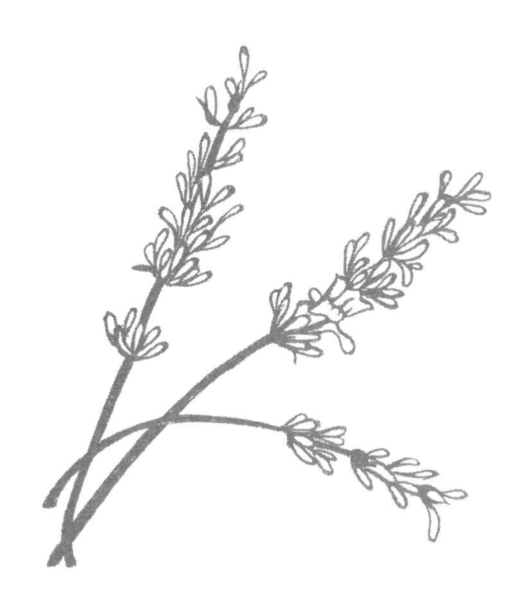

Champagne Rose Granita

Here's a new way to bring the classically romantic pairing of champagne and roses to your dinner table! This makes a great refreshing light dessert, or a sensual palate cleanser to serve between courses. Of course, with a little ingenuity, you can come up with some other ways to enjoy this simple, yet elegant ice!

½ cup sugar
½ cup spring water
1 tablespoon dried rose buds
1 inch piece of vanilla bean
1 cup champagne, chilled

Place an 8-inch square metal pan in the freezer to chill.
Place the first four ingredients into a small saucepan and simmer, stirring, until the sugar is melted and the flowers have wilted. Strain through a fine mesh sieve into a bowl and chill. Mix the champagne with the chilled syrup, pour into the metal pan and return to the freezer, uncovered. After about 1 hour, stir the slushy mixture vigorously with a fork. Continue to freeze, stirring every 30 minutes, until set, about 2–3 hours total. Scrape the granita with a fork and spoon into small serving dishes, or in hollowed out lemon halves. Garnish with a couple of fresh rose petals.

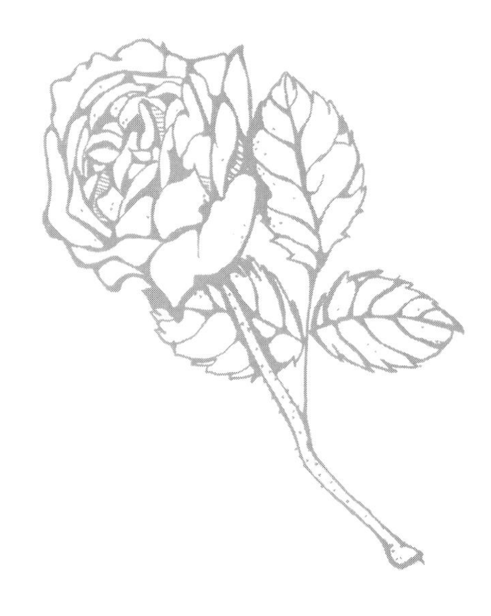

Jasmine Ice Cream

1 ½ cups milk
1 ½ cups cream
½ cup dried jasmine flowers
1 cup sugar
6 egg yolks

In a large saucepan, bring the milk, cream, and jasmine to a boil. Remove from heat and let steep for 20–30 minutes. Strain out the flowers through a sieve, pressing down on the flowers to extract all of the essences. Return the cream mixture to the pan, add ½ cup sugar and bring to a boil. Remove from heat. Beat the egg yolks with the remaining sugar. Temper the egg mixture by streaming in about ½ cup of the cream mixture, whisking constantly. Blend the egg mixture back into the remaining cream, and stir over low heat until thickened (do not boil). Process the mixture in an ice cream freezer.

The Indian god of love, Kama, used jasmine on the tips of his arrows to stimulate the sensual side of young lovers! The aromatherapeutic properties of jasmine as an aphrodisiac combine with the sultry palate feel of homemade ice cream to create a truly romantic dessert. The aroma of the flowers infusing the cream will perfume your mind with anticipation of things to come!

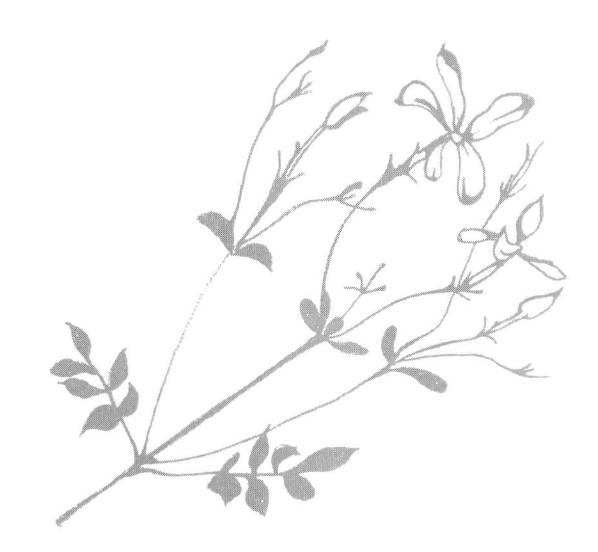

Rose Pudding

Is there anything that invokes feelings of romance more immediately than roses? The scent of rose is a favorite in scenting perfumes, and roses themselves are often the focal point of bridal bouquets. We hear tell that the petals from those bouquets are often strewn over the nuptual beddings to entice and invite further romance! We don't advise strewing this pudding about, but as a romantic dessert, it will surely help set the mood!

5 cups milk
1 cup whipping cream
½ cup rice flower
½ cup sugar
2 pods cardamom, crushed
3 tablespoons rose water*

Combine the rice flour and sugar and add to a saucepan containing the milk and cream. Slowly bring to a boil whisking vigorously for about 2 minutes, turn down to low. Add cardamom and continue stirring for one more minute. Remove from heat, and add rose water. Pour pudding into 6 individual ramekins. Allow to cool, and refrigerate for at least one hour.

**Rose water can be purchased at specialty food stores*

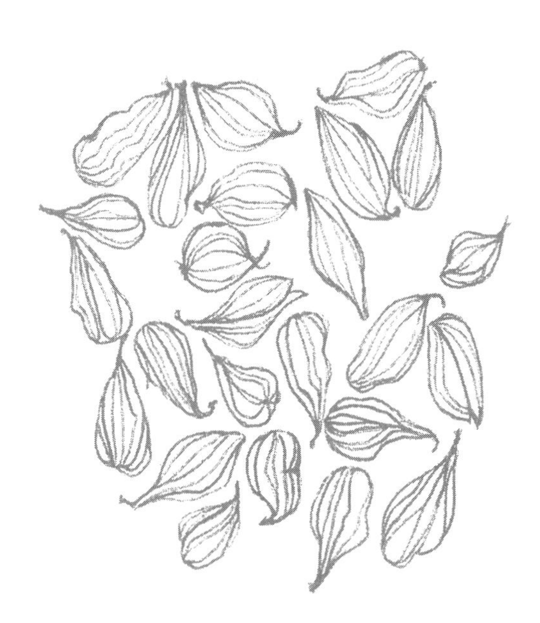

Lavender Crème Brûlée

2 cups heavy cream
2 teaspoons dried lavender flowers
¼ cup plus 4 tablespoons sugar
4 egg yolks
½ teaspoon vanilla extract

As if crème brûlée could be any more decadent, it is with the addition of lavender! Though this classic and sultry dessert is a favorite when dining in a fine restaurant, it is really very simple to create at home!

Preheat oven to 300°F. Have a kettle of simmering water ready.

In a saucepan, combine the cream, lavender and ¼ cup sugar and cook over medium-low heat for 8 minutes, stirring occasionally. Remove from heat. In a medium sized bowl, whisk the egg yolks and vanilla until the color is pale yellow and the yolks are smooth. Strain the cream mixture into the eggs, whisking constantly. Pour the mixture into four half-cup ramekins. Place the ramekins in a glass baking dish, and add the simmering water to come halfway up the sides of the ramekins. Bake for about 25 minutes, or until the custard is set. Remove the ramekins from the baking dish and let cool to room temperature. Just before serving, sprinkle the top of each ramekin with 1 tablespoon sugar. Use a kitchen torch to melt and brown the sugar until it forms a crust. In place of a kitchen torch, you can place the ramekins under a preheated broiler. Serve immediately.

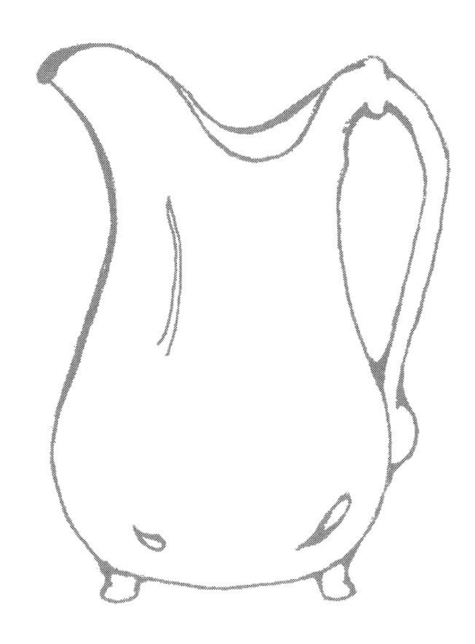

CHAPTER 3

RENEWING THE SOUL:
Recipes that Refresh and Invigorate

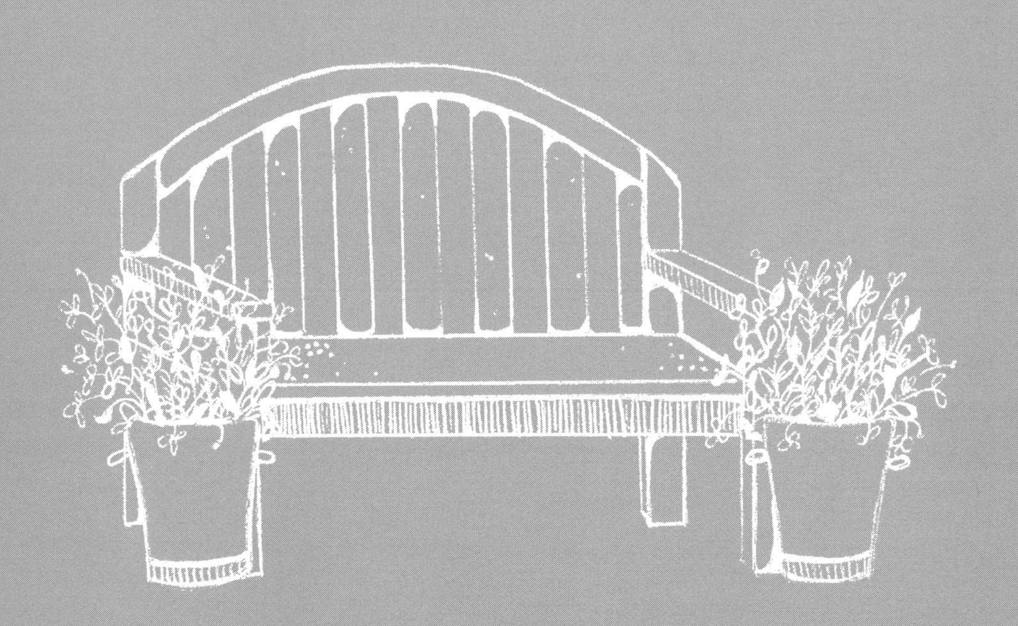

Enliven the Senses

Even those of us who love to cook can sometimes approach the kitchen with a groan. After a long, hard day at work (or at play, for that matter!), it can be difficult to get motivated to get in there and prepare a sensational meal. On these days, or any other day that you could use a little lift, turn to recipes that use herbs that are naturally invigorating! Rosemary immediately comes to mind, as do the essences of citrus fruits. But those are just the beginning! Read on to discover some fresh, new ways to bring a burst of energy into the kitchen—and into your body and spirit!

Carrot and Ginger Soup

Serves 6

During the Middle Ages, ginger was so popular in England that it became ingrained in the language as a verb, meaning to give life and zest. The use of ginger in the preparation and enjoyment of this soup will surely add some zest to your life!

2 tablespoons olive oil
1 onion, chopped
1 stalk lemongrass
⅓ cup grated fresh ginger root
3 cloves garlic, minced
2 star anise, optional
1 tablespoon black peppercorns
3 lbs carrots, peeled and chopped
7 cups vegetable stock
1 cup unsweetened coconut milk
crème fraîche, for garnish
chopped chive, for garnish
salt and cracked pepper to taste

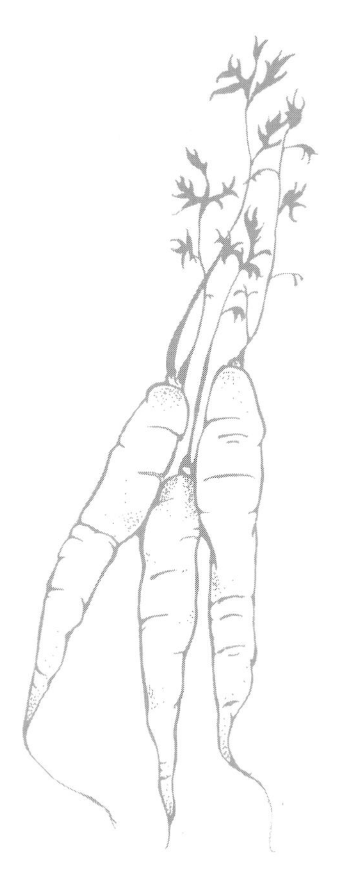

In a large stockpot, heat the oil over medium-high heat and sauté the onion, lemon grass and ginger for 5 minutes. Place the star anise and peppercorns onto a small piece of cheesecloth and tie into a bag. Place the carrots and peppercorn sachet in the pot, and add the vegetable stock. Cover, reduce heat to medium and cook for 30 minutes. Remove the lemongrass and pepper sachet. Puree the soup with a hand blender directly in the stockpot. Stir in the coconut milk, and salt to taste. Ladle the soup into serving bowls; add a dollop of crème fraîche, sprinkle with chopped chive, and cracked pepper.

South American Summer Salad

Serves 4–6

4 ears fresh corn (or 1 lb frozen kernels, thawed)
1 lb plum tomatoes, diced (keeping seeds and juices)
1 red onion, diced
1 chili, diced (use Santa Fe chili for a mild version, jalapeno for more heat)
1 cup minced cilantro
juice of ½ lemon
juice of ½ lime
½ teaspoon tabasco, or to taste
¾ cup red wine vinegar
½ cup canola oil
freshly ground sea salt and black pepper, to taste

In Chile and Argentina, this marinated salad is a summer staple! The fresh flavors of tomato and corn are spiked to another level with citrus, cilantro, and chilies. It's great served as a first course with some crusty bread to scoop up the salad, or as a side dish alongside a sizzling serving of grilled chicken or fish! On a refreshing scale of 1 to 10, we definitely give this a 10!

If using fresh corn, lightly steam the ears, and cut the kernels from the cobs. Place into a large glass or wood bowl. Add the remaining ingredients and combine well. Let your taste buds be your guide when adding chilies—even the same variety of chili varies in heat quotient from chili to chili! Let the salad marinate for at least one hour before serving.

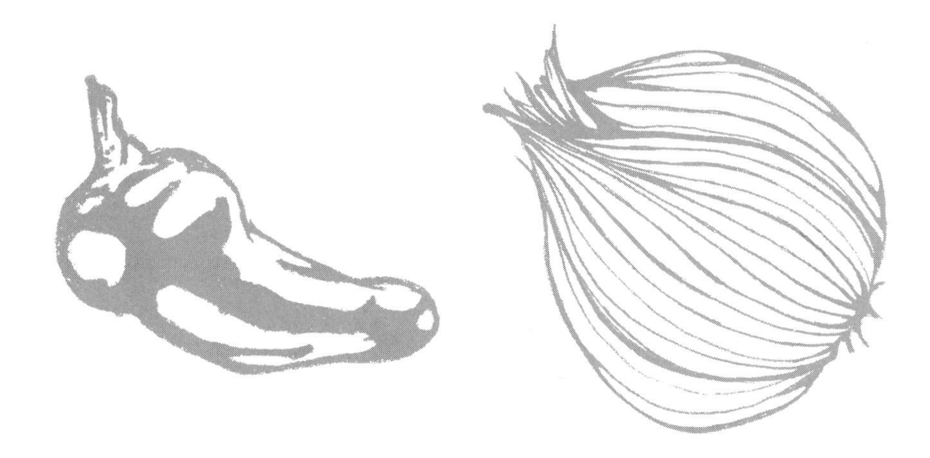

Minty Taboulleh

Serves 4

The combination of citrus, mint, and parsley just screams refreshing! It pairs perfectly with our Indian Chicken with ginger and cumin.

8 green onions
1 teaspoon oil

1 cup couscous
1 cup water

4 cups chopped parsley
½ cup chopped mint
3 plum tomatoes, seeded and chopped

4 tablespoons lemon juice
4 tablespoons lime juice
1 garlic clove, crushed
¾ cup olive oil
salt and pepper

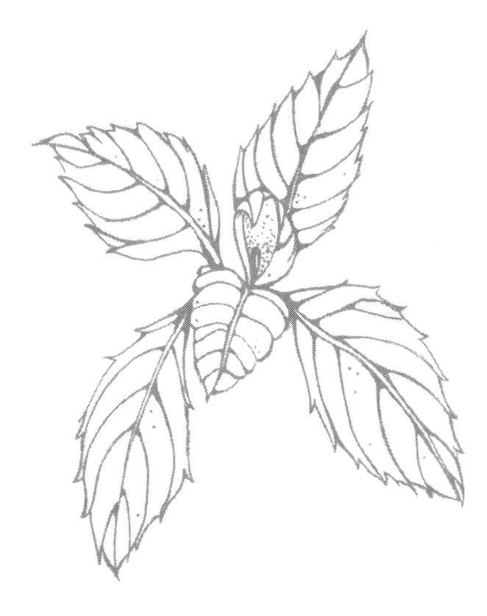

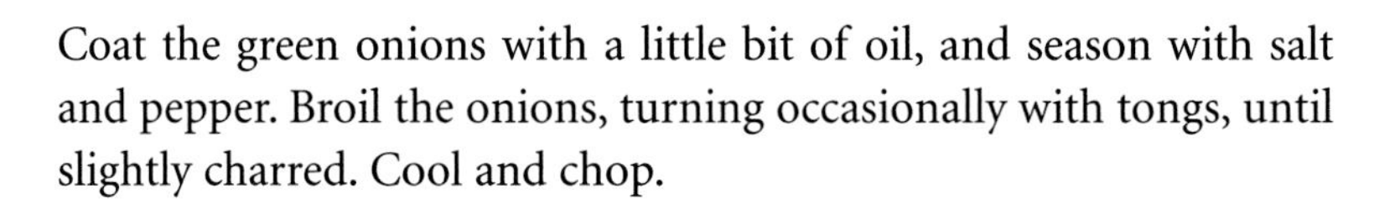

Coat the green onions with a little bit of oil, and season with salt and pepper. Broil the onions, turning occasionally with tongs, until slightly charred. Cool and chop.

In a small saucepan, bring the water to a boil. Add the couscous, stir, cover and remove from heat. Let stand for 5 minutes. Fluff the couscous with a fork. Let cool completely.

In a large bowl, combine the parsley, mint and tomatoes. Add the green onions and couscous. Whisk together the lemon, lime garlic, oil, and salt and pepper to taste. Pour over the parsley mixture and combine well.

Rosemary and Goat Cheese Tart

Serves 6 as a first course

1 ¾ cups flour
3 tablespoons blue cheese, crumbled
7 tablespoons butter, chilled
4 tablespoons ice water

¼ cup plus 1 tablespoon heavy cream
12 oz goat cheese
2 ¼ tablespoons chopped rosemary leaves
2 tablespoons lemon zest
salt and pepper

The scent of rosemary has long been attributed to improving memory. In ancient Greece, students wore garlands of rosemary to help them retain knowledge! To add some great color to this fragrant tart, slice up some roasted red and yellow peppers to fan over the finished tart.

Place the flour in a mixing bowl. Add the blue cheese and butter and work with your fingers to make a crumbly dough. Add the water, 1 tablespoon at a time, until the pastry comes together as a smooth ball. Wrap in plastic and refrigerate for 2–3 hours.

Meanwhile, in a food processor, mix the cream, goat cheese, rosemary, lemon zest and salt and pepper to taste. Wrap in plastic and chill for 2 hours.

Preheat oven to 350°F. Remove dough from refrigerator and roll out into a 10-inch circle. Press into an 8-inch pie pan, and prick the bottom with a fork. Cover the bottom with foil and cover with pie weights or dried beans to keep the crust from rising. Bake the crust for 15 minutes, or until golden brown. Remove the foil and weights and cool for 5 minutes. Spread the goat cheese mixture over the crust and bake for 35 minutes.

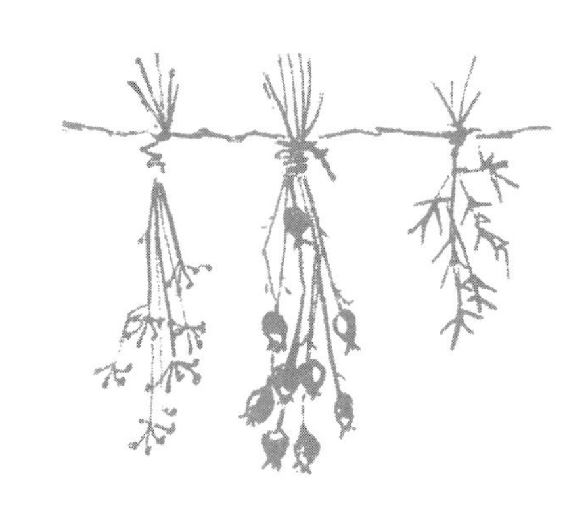

Eggplant Rolls with Feta and Mint

Serves 4–6 as a first course

The pairing of refreshing mint with sassy feta cheese is sure to enliven the taste buds! The addition of a little cinnamon in the bell pepper sauce heightens the experience even further! These rolls are great as a first course, or served beside a simple grilled fish or chicken.

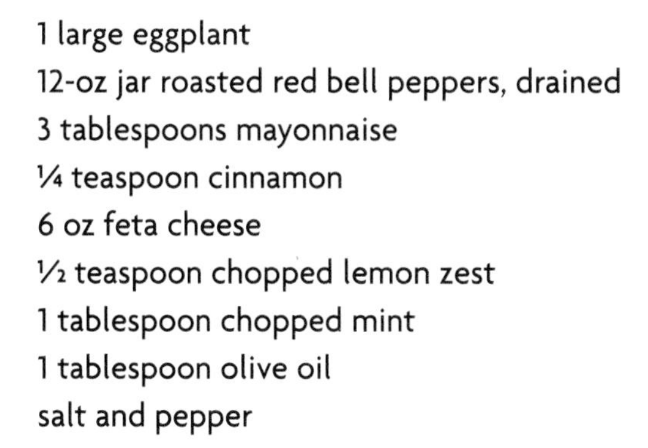

1 large eggplant
12-oz jar roasted red bell peppers, drained
3 tablespoons mayonnaise
¼ teaspoon cinnamon
6 oz feta cheese
½ teaspoon chopped lemon zest
1 tablespoon chopped mint
1 tablespoon olive oil
salt and pepper

Slice the eggplant into ¼ inch rounds. Pick out the twelve largest rounds and reserve the rest for another use. Place the rounds in a colander and sprinkle generously with salt. Let the eggplant "sweat" for 30 minutes (this process removes the bitter taste from the eggplant and also reduces its tendency to soak up oil). Rinse the eggplant well and pat dry. Heat a ridged grill pan over medium-high heat. Brush lightly with olive oil. Grill the eggplant until nicely marked on both sides. Remove to a working surface, such as a large cutting board.

Preheat oven to 375°F. In a mixing bowl, blend together the feta, lemon zest, mint, and salt and pepper to taste. Form about 1 tablespoon of the mixture into a log with your hands, place onto the lower third of an eggplant round and roll to enclose the cheese. Place on a baking sheet. Continue with the remaining rounds. Bake for about 5 minutes, or until the cheese has just started to melt. In a food processor or blender, puree the roasted red peppers with the mayonnaise and cinnamon until smooth. Season with salt and pepper. Serve the rolls with a dollop of the bell pepper sauce.

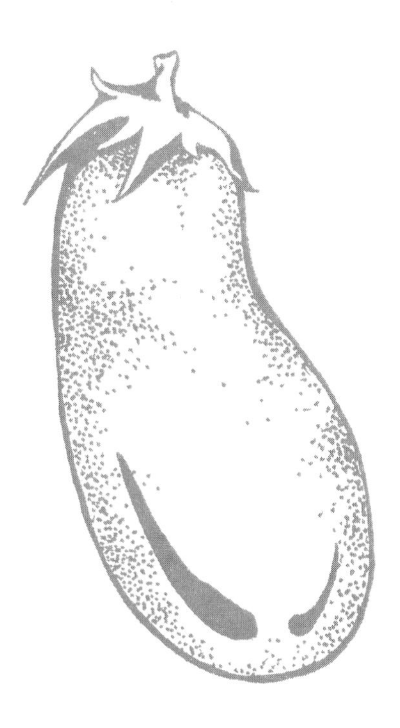

Chilean Seabass with Rosemary Butter

Serves 2

¾ lb Chilean seabass
4 tablespoons olive oil
¼ cup chopped onion
1 ½ cups chopped leek
¾ cup chopped mushrooms
bouquet garni*
1 cup dry white wine
½ cup water
3 six-inch branches rosemary
6 tablespoons butter, chilled

Rosemary has long been considered a good-luck plant, and is a symbol of love and loyalty. So it's no surprise that the Greeks would include a few sprigs of rosemary in bridal bouquets. Ancient lore continues that if once planted those sprigs took root and flourished, that the woman would rule the house! (Amazingly, this notion was considered vulgar by some men, who would try to sabotage the plants!)

Heat the olive oil in a skillet over medium-high heat. Sauté the onion, leek, mushrooms and bouquet garni for 5 minutes. Add the wine, water and rosemary, cover and cook for 20 minutes. Strain through a sieve, and return the liquid to the pan. Bring the liquid to a simmer and poach the fish for 10 minutes or until opaque. Remove the fish to a plate, cover and keep warm. Bring the poaching liquid to a boil and reduce to half its volume. Lower the heat to medium and whisk in the butter, one piece at a time, and cook until slightly thickened. Spoon the sauce over the fish and serve.

**Bouquet garni is a bundle of aromatics—typically thyme, parsley, and bay leaf—tied together in a cheesecloth. In this case you can omit the cheesecloth since the sauce will be strained.*

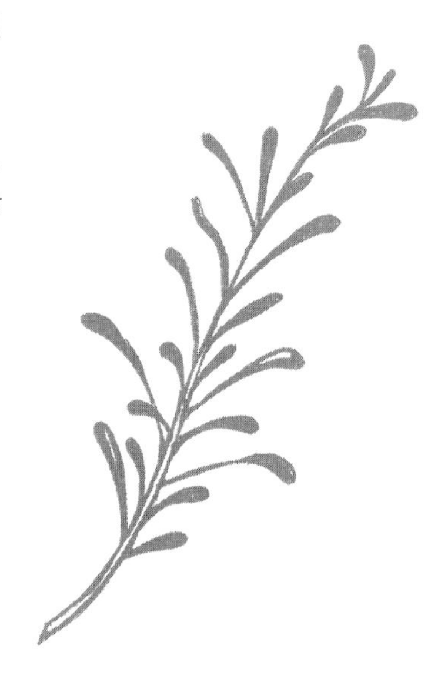

Chipotle-Mint Game Hen

Serves 2

Chipotles are dried smoked jalapeno peppers, which have a wonderful depth of flavor without being too hot to handle! They are offered canned in "adobo" sauce in many markets, but we prefer to use the dried variety—if it's not on your market shelves it can be ordered from spice suppliers (see appendix). The addition of some spunky mint and zesty lemon really make this bird sing!

1 cup fresh mint leaves, loosely packed
1 tablespoon chipotle powder, or to taste
1 lemon
1 ½ lb game hen, rinsed and patted dry

Preheat oven to 450°F. Place the hen in a roasting pan. Squeeze the lemon over the game hen, and place one lemon half inside the cavity. Loosen the skin over the hen breasts and stuff some of the mint leaves between the skin and the flesh. Put the rest of the mint inside the cavity. Sprinkle the chipotle over the outside of the hen to dust evenly, and use the remainder to season the inside of the cavity. Roast the hen for 15 minutes. Baste with the pan juices and continue roasting for an additional 10 minutes, or until the juices run clear. Remove from oven and let rest 10 minutes. Split the bird in half and spoon the pan juices over the meat.

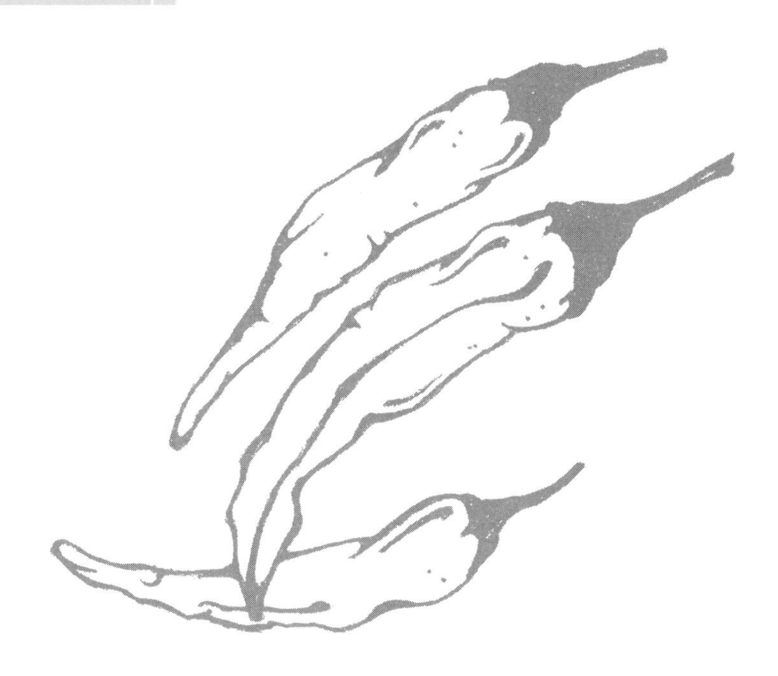

Fava Bean Ragout

Serves 4

5 whole garlic cloves
1 lb plum tomatoes, quartered
2 tablespoons olive oil
salt and pepper

3 cups fava beans*
½ cup chicken or vegetable stock
½ cup dry white wine
½ teaspoon cumin
½ teaspoon ground coriander
¼ teaspoon ground cardamom
1 tablespoon minced fresh oregano
1 tablespoon tomato paste

Fava beans are nutritious, hearty, and eager to be infused with flavorful herbs and spices. This lively version is great on its own for a vegetarian entrée, or as a side dish along side poultry or fish. If you're a fan of "The Silence of the Lambs", you might want to serve it with a nice Chianti!

Preheat oven to 425°F. Place the garlic and tomatoes on a baking sheet, drizzle with the olive oil and season with salt and pepper. Roast in the oven for 30 minutes. Remove from oven and set aside.

In a 2-qt saucepan, cook the fava beans in the stock over medium heat, covered, for 30 minutes, or until the beans are soft but not mushy. Add the roasted tomatoes and garlic, wine, spices and the oregano, and cook uncovered for an additional 10–15 minutes. Stir in the tomato paste, and cook until thickened, about 5–8 minutes.

**If using fresh fava beans, simply remove the skins from the beans (note that cooking time may be less than 30 minutes). If using dried beans, soak overnight in a bowl covered with 3 inches of water. Drain and remove skins the next day.*

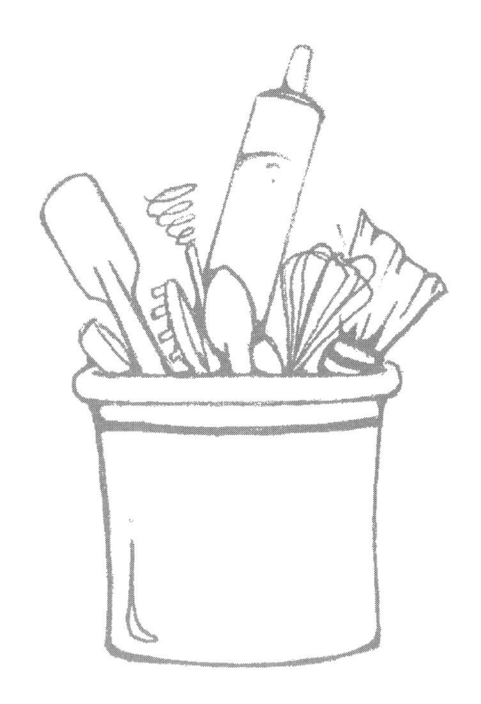

Ginger Chicken with Shiitake Mushrooms

Serves 4–6

Don't be intimidated by the amount of ginger called for in this dish! Though the aroma and flavor of the ginger are strikingly invigorating, they are not overpowering!

4 tablespoons canola oil
2 lb boneless chicken breast, diced
8 oz shiitake mushrooms, sliced
2 garlic cloves, minced
¼ cup minced ginger root
1 cup heavy cream
salt and pepper to taste
4 tablespoons sliced chive

1 lb pasta

In a large skillet, heat the oil over medium-high heat. Add the chicken and sauté until lightly browned. Reduce heat to medium, add the mushrooms, garlic, ginger, and salt and pepper to taste (go a little heavy on the pepper!). Saute for 3–5 minutes. Pour in the cream, cover and cook for 8–10 minutes.

In a large pot of boiling salted water, cook the pasta until al dente. Drain and transfer to a large serving bowl. Pour the chicken mixture over the pasta and toss until well combined. Sprinkle with the chives, and serve.

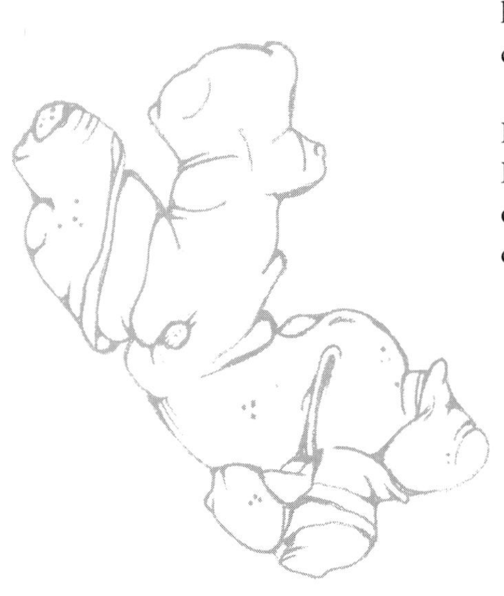

Herbed Pork Chops with Port Reduction

Serves 2

2 boneless 1-inch thick center cut pork chops (about 1 lb)
3 garlic cloves, minced
1 tablespoon minced rosemary
1 teaspoon minced thyme
salt and pepper to taste
2 teaspoons olive oil

1 tablespoon olive oil
½ cup sliced mushrooms
1 tablespoon flour
¼ cup chicken stock
¾ cup port
salt and pepper to taste

Rosemary was often used as incense in religious ceremonies as well as in magical spells to ward off evil spirits and bad dreams. The scent of this savory pork will surely work magic on your soul!

Grind the garlic and herbs together with the oil in a mortar and pestle until well combined (can use a mini-food processor in place of mortar and pestle). Spread the herb mixture over both sides of the chops and let sit, refrigerated, for 20–30 minutes. Preheat a nonstick skillet (preferably a ridged grill pan) over medium-high heat. Add the chops and sear on both sides until nicely browned. Reduce heat to medium, and continue cooking until the pink just disappears, about 8–10 minutes.

While the chops are cooking, heat the olive oil over medium-high heat in a small saucepan. Add the mushrooms and cook, stirring occasionally, for 5 minutes. Sprinkle the flour over the mushrooms and stir until coated. Pour in the stock and the port, bring to a boil, and reduce to half its volume. The sauce should be thick and glossy. Season with salt and pepper.

To serve, place a swirl of the port reduction on each plate, and top with a pork chop. Garnish with a sprig of fresh rosemary, and pass extra sauce at the table.

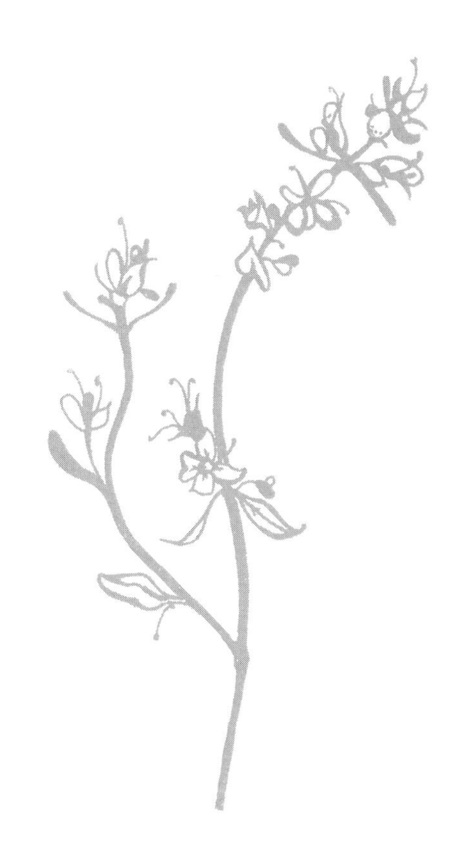

Cumin Coriander Couscous with Turkey Meatballs

Serves 4–6

Cumin and coriander are the staple spices of Morrocan cooking. They are delightfully fragrant and will fill your kitchen and your senses with an exotic atmosphere!

2 lbs ground turkey
3 slices white bread
½ cup milk
3 tablespoons ground coriander
1 ½ tablespoons ground cumin
3 tablespoons canola oil
1 onion, chopped
1 ½ cups water
¾ cup golden raisins
¾ cup garbanzo beans, canned, drained
salt and pepper

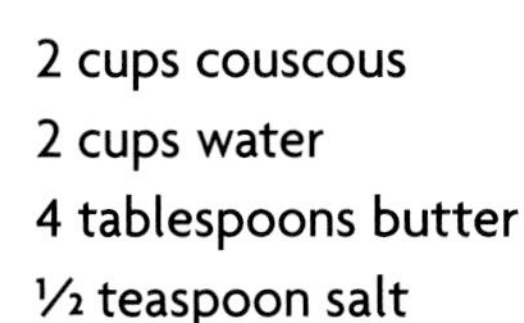

2 cups couscous
2 cups water
4 tablespoons butter
½ teaspoon salt

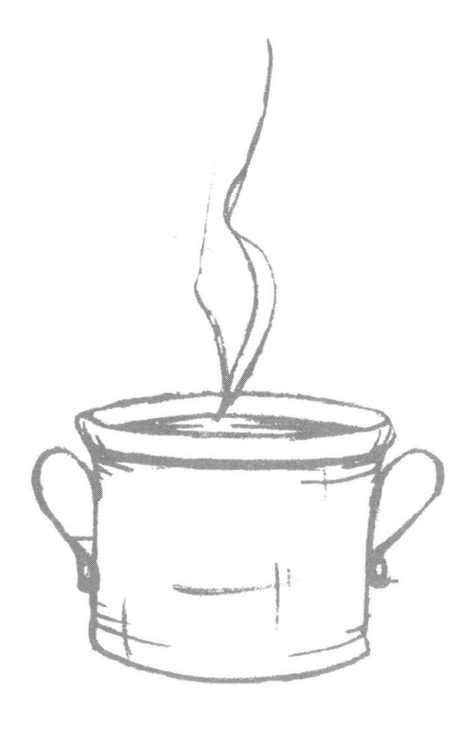

Trim the crusts off the bread and soak in milk in a large bowl for 5 minutes. Add the ground turkey, coriander, cumin, salt and pepper to taste, and mix well. Form into 1 inch round meatballs. In a large skillet, heat the oil over medium/high heat. Add the meatballs and cook until browned, about 5 minutes. Lower the heat to medium, add the water, onions, and raisins, and cook for 20 minutes.

While the meatballs are cooking, make the couscous. In a large saucepan, bring the water, butter, and salt to a boil. Add the couscous, stir well, cover and remove from heat. Let stand for 5 minutes. Fluff with a fork before serving.

Spoon the couscous into serving bowls, make a well in the center, and ladle in the meatballs.

Penne with Smoked Salmon in Lemon-Vodka Cream

Serves 2

½ lb penne
1 shallot, minced
½ cup chopped lemon verbena
¾ cup vodka
½ cup crème fraîche
1 cup cream
zest of 1 lemon
½ lb smoked salmon fillet
salt and white pepper

Lemon verbena is a favored scent for perfumes, as it carries a clean and refreshing aroma. In Spain it was used to impart its lively scent to finger bowls for cleansing the hands between courses. We find lemon verbena to add a lively twist to the classic salmon pasta with vodka cream.

Bring water and 1 teaspoon salt to boil in a 2½ quart saucepan. Cook the pasta until just al dente, about 8 minutes. Strain in a colander and rinse with warm water. Rinse out the pan, and towel dry. Mix the shallot, verbena, and vodka in the saucepan, and bring to a vigorous simmer. Add the crème fraîche and the cream and simmer until thickened. Add the lemon zest, salmon, pasta and salt and pepper to taste, and cook until just heated through. Serve in pasta bowls with a little lemon zest and fresh verbena as garnish.

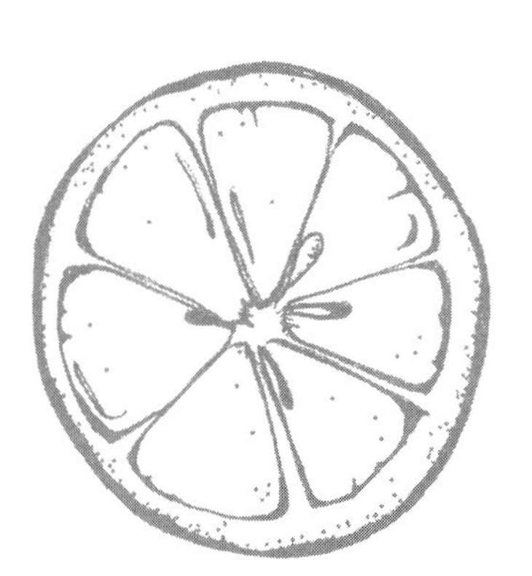

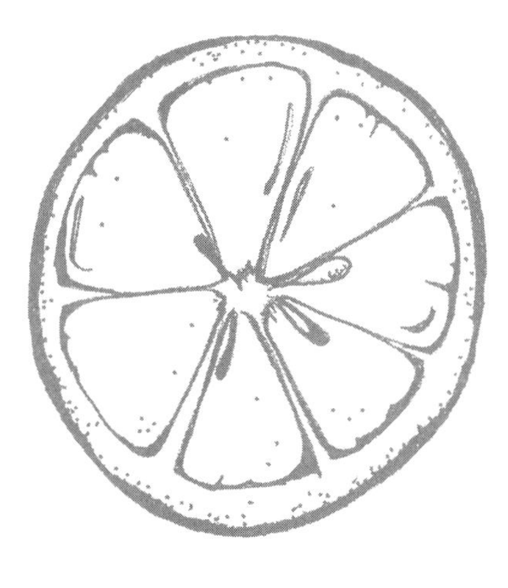

Roasted Rosemary Chicken with Caramelized Apples

Serves 4

Rosemary is renowned for its stimulating properties, as anyone who has ever delighted in its scent will attest! The reaction is not only emotional, but physical as well—the scent of rosemary actually stimulates the mind as it increases the brain's beta waves!

1 whole 4–5 lb chicken
3 tablespoons chopped rosemary, plus a few whole sprigs
1 tablespoon thyme
2 tablespoons kosher salt
6 tablespoons butter, softened

4 apples, quartered and cored
½ cup white wine vinegar
¼ cup sugar
4 tablespoons butter, cut into small pieces, chilled
salt and pepper

Preheat oven to 400°F. Mix together the butter, rosemary, thyme and salt. Rinse the chicken under cold water and pat dry. Rub the chicken all over with the rosemary mixture. Put the whole rosemary sprigs into the cavity of the bird. Place the chicken in a roasting pan and bake for 15 minutes per pound, or until the juices run clear.

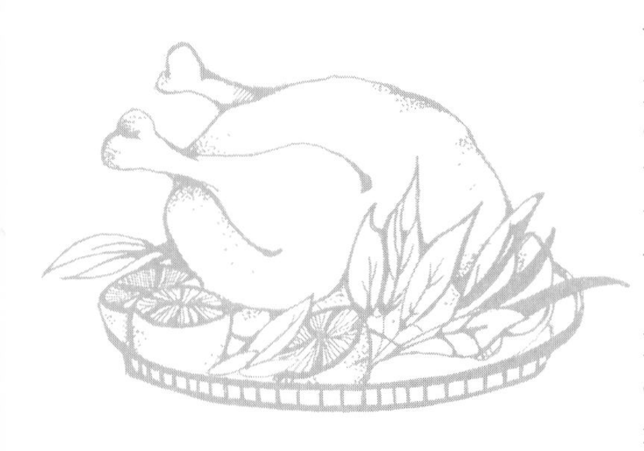

While the chicken is cooking, mix the vinegar and sugar in a frying pan. Cook over medium heat for 5 minutes. Add the apples and cook for 5 minutes. Turn the apples and cook for another 5 minutes, until golden. Stir in the butter, a few pieces at a time, and cook until the sauce coats the back of a spoon. Add salt and pepper to taste.

Remove the chicken from the oven and let rest for 10 minutes. Carve into serving pieces. Arrange the chicken and apples on serving plates and drizzle with the sauce.

Roasted Salmon with Cinnamon and Cumin

Serves 4

4 salmon fillets (6–8 oz each)
¼ cup orange juice
1 tablespoon lemon Juice
2 tablespoons grated orange zest
¾ teaspoon cumin
¼ teaspoon cinnamon
2 tablespoons brown sugar
salt and pepper

Your taste buds will surely come alive with the wonderful flavors in this dish! Let the spicy aromas work their magic to invigorate the senses and stimulate the appetite!

Combine orange & lemon juice and pour over salmon in a marinating dish. Refrigerate for up to 2 hours.

Preheat oven to 400°F. Combine sugar, orange rind, cumin, cinnamon, and salt and pepper in a small bowl. Remove fish from the marinating dish and place in an oiled baking dish. Rub the sugar mixture over both sides of the salmon and bake in the oven for approximately 10–15 minutes, until the salmon is just opaque.

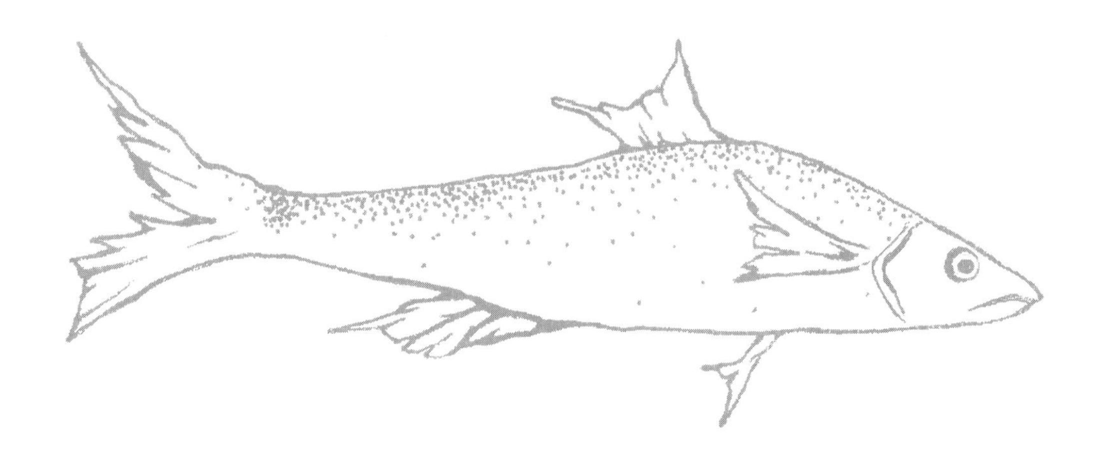

Rosemary-Pine Nut Crusted Pork Loin

Serves 4

The herb rub for this pork is so tantalizing and aromatic, that you might find yourself sneaking bites before it even gets on the roast! Just wait till you smell the aromas as it cooks in the oven—wow!

⅓ cup fresh rosemary leaves
1 cup pine nuts
1 large garlic clove
2 tablespoons olive oil
salt and pepper to taste

1 lb pork tenderloin

½ cup white wine
1 teaspoon cornstarch

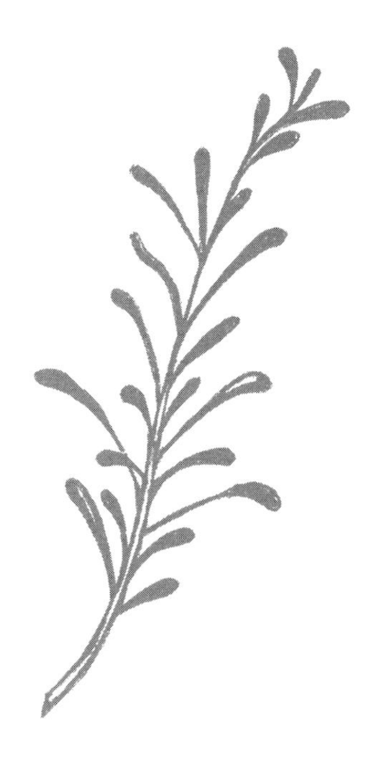

Preheat oven to 400°F. In a food processor, blend the rosemary, pine nuts, garlic and salt and pepper. With the motor running, stream in the oil and process until the mixture forms into a ball. Rub the pork loin all over with the herb paste and place into the pan. Bake for 20 minutes or until internal temperature reaches 150°F (if you don't have a meat thermometer, buy one! They are inexpensive and indispensable to ensure proper cooking times). Remove the pork to a cutting board and let rest. Pour the pan juices into a saucepan, scraping any brown bits into the saucepan. Bring to a boil, add the wine and reduce for 5–8 minutes. Dissolve the cornstarch in a small amount of cold water and add to the sauce. Bring to a boil and stir until thickened. Slice the pork and serve drizzled with some of the sauce. Pass additional sauce at the table.

Spiced Shrimp Sauté

Serves 2

12 jumbo shrimp (16-20 count), peeled and deveined
1 tablespoon lime juice

1 tablespoon cardamom
2 teaspoons allspice
1 tablespoon garlic powder
¼ teaspoon cinnamon
¼ teaspoon cayenne

1 tablespoon canola oil
1 small onion, chopped
½ cup chopped red bell pepper
1 cup sliced mushrooms

Cardamom, the star of this spice combination, is prized as a stimulant as well as serving as a digestive aid and a breath freshener! What more could one ask from a spice? Oh, yeah—explosively great flavor, which cardamom delivers as well, especially in combination with the other spices in this dish! Save any remaining spice mix to add some spark to rice dishes and couscous.

Toss the shrimp with the lime juice in a glass bowl and set aside. In a small bowl, combine all of the spices, mixing well. Set aside.

Heat the oil over medium-high heat in a medium skillet and sauté the onion for 5 minutes. Add the bell pepper and mushrooms and continue cooking for 8–10 minutes. Dredge each shrimp in the spice mix and add to the sauté pan. Cook over high heat, stirring frequently, until the shrimp are just cooked through, about 3 minutes. Serve over couscous or rice.

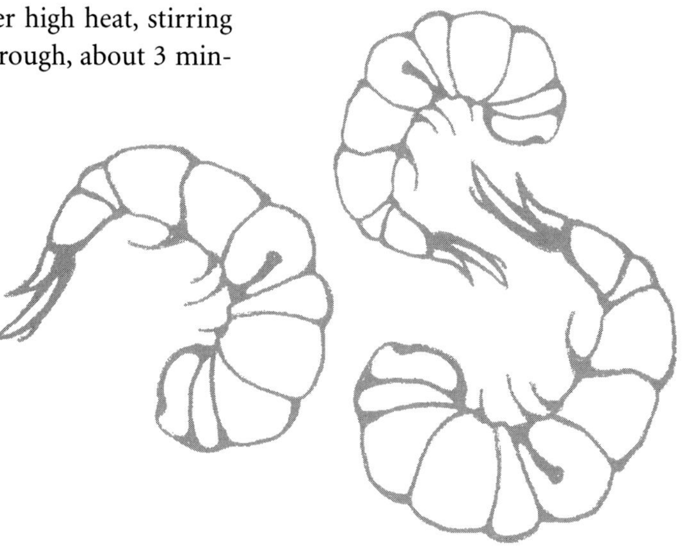

Tilapia with Sauce Provencal

Serves 4

A friendly warning before you make this recipe: it will not do well on a first date! The sauce is infused with plenty of garlic, which in combination with the fresh herbs will leave your senses sizzling!

8 tilapia filets (can substitute sole)
1 tomato
1 cup chopped basil
4 leaves lemon verbena, chopped
1 shallot, minced
1 garlic clove, minced
½ teaspoon balsamic vinegar
¾ cup olive oil, plus 1 tablespoon olive oil

Bring a small pan of water to a boil and have a bowl of ice water ready. Parboil the tomato for about 45 seconds, and transfer it to the ice water. Remove the peel, seed, and chop. In a mixing bowl toss the tomato with the basil, lemon verbena, shallot, and garlic. Add the vinegar and oil, and season with salt and pepper to taste.

Heat 1 tablespoon olive oil in a skillet and sauté the fish until it is opaque. Plate 2 filets per person, and top with the sauce.

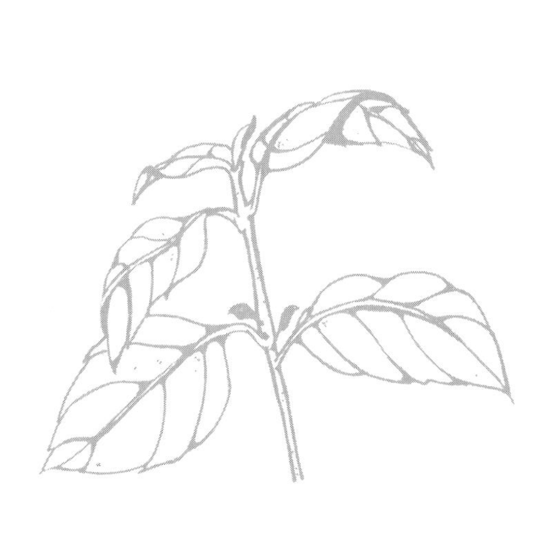

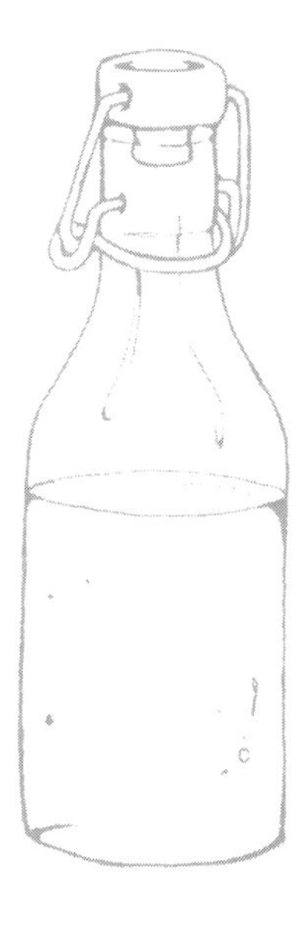

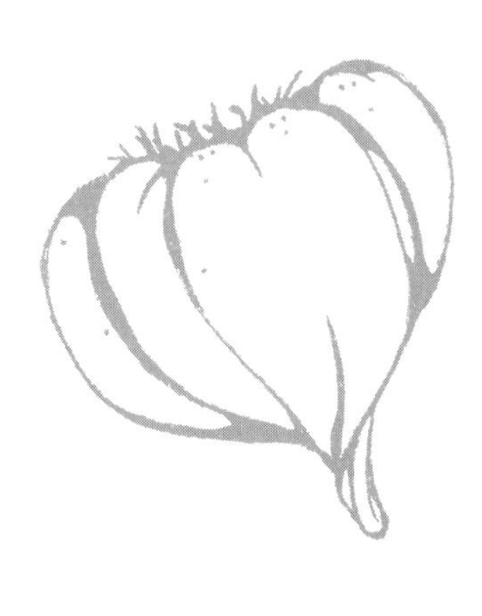

Indian Chicken with Ginger and Cumin

Serves 4

2 cups yogurt
6 garlic cloves, minced
3 tablespoons minced ginger
2 tablespoons cumin
4 boneless, skinless chicken breast halves
salt and pepper

Indian spices are wonderful for creating a lively and simple chicken dish that will enliven your senses!

Combine the yogurt, garlic, ginger and cumin. Season the chicken breasts with salt and pepper. Pierce several times with a fork. Pour two-thirds of the yogurt mixture over the chicken and marinate, covered, for at least 3 hours, or overnight.

Preheat oven to 375°F. Place the chicken breasts on a baking sheet and cook in the oven for 15–20 minutes, depending on the thickness of the chicken. Serve over jasmine rice, using the remaining yogurt mixture as a dipping sauce.

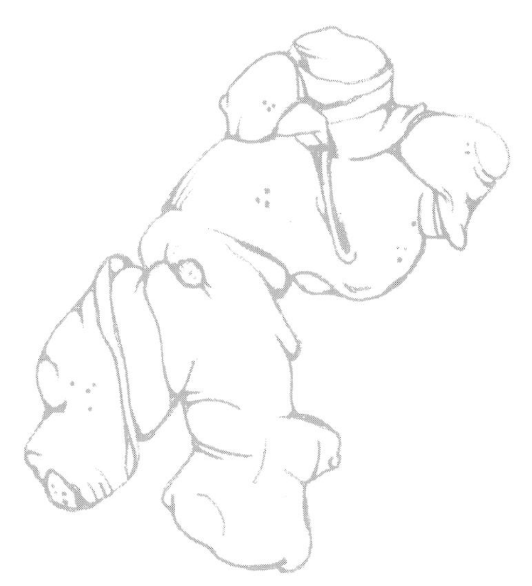

Rosemary Roasted Vegetables with Bulgur Pilaf

Serves 4–6

This is a healthy and hearty one-dish meal that well serves the attributes of rosemary as an herb of friendship and love. It's a great way to infuse the house with the stimulating scent of rosemary, and makes for a very fragrant and warming meal in the fall or winter. One whiff of these veggies roasting will get people running to the kitchen!

2 cups bulgur
4 cups water

12 garlic cloves
1 onion, cut into wedges
2 carrots, sliced
4 plum tomatoes, cut in half
1 Japanese eggplant, cubed
1 red bell pepper, chopped
½ small butternut squash, peeled and cubed
¼ cup chopped rosemary
olive oil
1 can garbanzo beans
1 lemon
salt and pepper

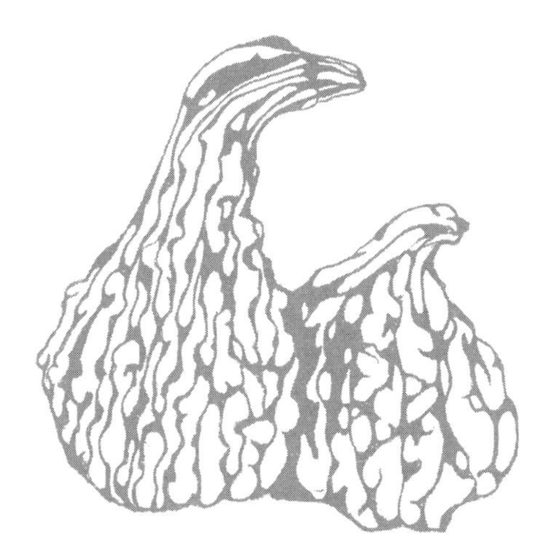

In a medium saucepan, combine the bulgur and water. Bring to a boil. Cover, reduce heat, and simmer for 20–25 minutes, or until all of the water is absorbed. Remove from heat.

Preheat oven to 400°F. Arrange all of the vegetables, except the garbanzo beans, on a large baking sheet. Sprinkle with half of the rosemary. Drizzle generously with the oil, and toss lightly with your hands to coat the veggies. Roast the vegetables in the oven for 45–60 minutes, stirring occasionally. Season with salt and pepper.

In a large bowl, combine the bulgur, roasted veggies, garbanzo beans, and remaining rosemary. Squeeze the lemon over the mixture, and toss well.

Rosemary Strata

Serves 6

3 tablespoons canola oil
2 leeks, cut into half-inch slices
2 onions, diced
10 eggs
2 cups heavy cream
1 cup whole milk
1 ½ teaspoon salt
1 teaspoon pepper
1 baguette, sliced into 1-inch rounds, and lightly toasted
½ lb Monterey Jack cheese
½ lb Swiss cheese
¼ cup finely minced rosemary (*note:* mince it really well!)

This is the perfect dish to prepare for a brunch, as all of the work (including clean-up!) is done the night before. When your guests arrive, they will be immediately uplifted from the aroma of the fresh rosemary and will be amazed at your spotless kitchen!

Heat the oil in a saucepan over medium heat. Add the leek and onion and cook until translucent, about 5 minutes. In a large bowl, mix the eggs, cream, milk, salt and pepper. Place half of the baguette slices in the bottom of a 9 x 13 glass baking dish. Sprinkle with half of the onion mixture, half of the Monterey Jack, half of the Swiss, and half of the rosemary. Make a second layer with the bread, veggies, cheeses, and rosemary. Pour the cream mixture slowly over the bread, and cover tightly with plastic wrap or foil. Refrigerate overnight.

Preheat oven to 375°F. Bake the strata, uncovered, for 40–50 minutes, or until the cheese is bubbling and golden brown. Remove from oven and let sit for 10 minutes before serving.

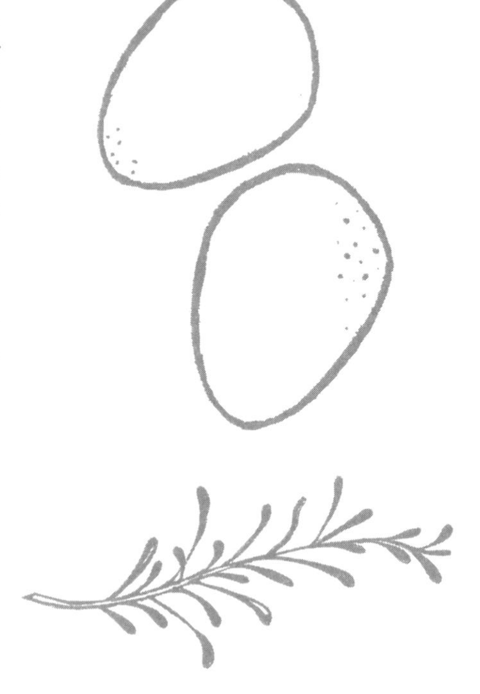

Green Beans with Spiced Candied Walnuts

Serves 4

Sweet and spicy walnuts enliven sautéed green beans to a new dimension! Go ahead and turn up the heat with extra cayenne if you really want to fire up your senses!

1 cup walnuts
6 tablespoons brown sugar
2 tablespoons water
1 teaspoon cayenne pepper

1 tablespoon canola oil
1 tablespoon butter
2 shallots, sliced
1 lb green beans, trimmed
½ teaspoon black pepper

Combine the sugar, water, and cayenne in a small saucepan and heat until the sugar is dissolved. Bring to a boil, add the walnuts, and stir until well-coated and the foam has subsided. Pour out onto a sheet of waxed paper, separating the nuts, and allow to cool.

Heat the oil and butter in a large skillet over medium-high heat and sauté the shallots for 3 minutes. Add the beans and black pepper and sauté for 5 minutes. Toss in the walnuts and continue to sauté for about 3 minutes, or until the beans are just crisp-tender.

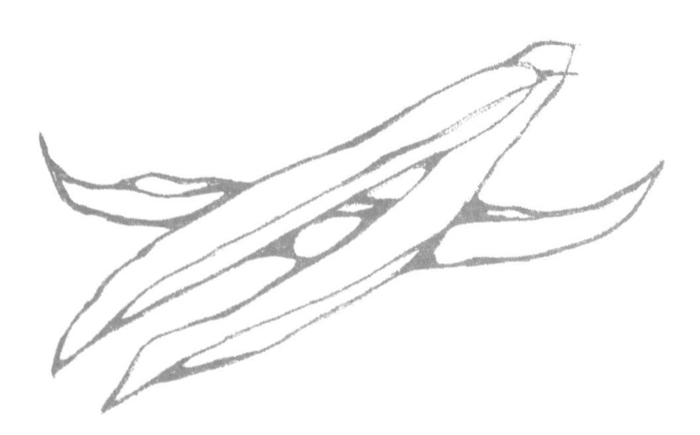

Citrus-Ginger Cheesecake

1 ¾ cups graham cracker crumbs
⅔ cup brown sugar
¼ cup melted butter
2 ½ cups ricotta cheese
1 tablespoon finely minced lemon zest
1 tablespoon finely minced orange zest
½ cup sugar
½ cup sour cream
3 eggs
½ tablespoon grated ginger

Citrus . . . ginger . . . cheesecake. Are you salivating yet? If not, you will as the aromas of this great combination attack your olfactory senses! Your taste buds will jump for joy upon the first (but certainly not last) sensational bite!

Preheat oven to 350°F. In a bowl, combine the graham cracker crumbs, brown sugar, and melted butter and mix well. Press the mixture evenly into the bottom of a 9-inch springform pan.

In a separate bowl, mix the ricotta, citrus zests, sugar, sour cream, eggs, and ginger. Beat until smooth. Pour the mixture over the crust and bake for 50 minutes, or until a knife inserted in the middle comes out clean. Remove from oven and let rest for one hour at room temperature, then chill for 2–3 hours before serving.

Citrus Soufflés with Grand Marnier

Soufflés are not as difficult as you might think! They take a little forethought, but follow our instructions and you will have a delightful (and impressive!) outcome. This recipe has served us well in serving up a fruitful closing to an invigorating evening!

¼ cup butter, plus additional for preparing ramekins
1/4 cup flour
1 cup milk
½ cup sugar
4 tablespoons fresh orange juice
2 tablespoons fresh lemon juice
1 ½ teaspoon chopped orange zest
1 teaspoon chopped lemon zest
4 egg yolks
5 egg whites
1 tablespoon Grand Marnier, plus extra for serving

Preheat oven to 375°F. Have a kettle of simmering water ready. Prepare six ¾ cup ramekins by coating the inside and upper rim thoroughly with butter.

In a saucepan, melt the butter over medium heat. Sprinkle in the flour, mix thoroughly and cook, stirring, for 3 minutes. Whisk in the milk and heat, stirring until it just comes to a boil. Add 6 tablespoons of the sugar, the juices and zests, return to a boil, and then remove from heat. In a small bowl, whisk the egg yolks until light yellow and uniform in consistency. Once the base white sauce has cooled slightly, drop a few tablespoons, one at a time, into the egg yolk whisking constantly to temper the yolks. Return the yolk mixture to the base sauce and whisk until incorporated. Stir in the Grand Marnier. *Note:* This can be prepared several hours in advance. Cover and set aside until ready to finish the preparation.

Place the egg whites unto a very clean bowl of a stand mixer. Beat the whites to medium stiff peaks. Add the remaining 2 tablespoons sugar and continue beating until the peaks are stiff but not dry. Stir about 1/4 of the whites into the base sauce. Transfer the base sauce into the bowl with the remaining whites and fold gently to combine. Pour the mixture into the ramekins, filling about 3/4 full. Place the ramekins in a glass baking dish, such that the ramekins are not touching one another. Set the dish on the oven rack, and carefully pour the simmering water into the bottom of the pan to create a bath that reaches halfway up the sides of the ramekins. Bake the soufflés until puffy and golden brown, about 15 minutes. Remove the ramekins to small dessert plates, and serve with a couple of madeleines or shortbread cookies and a small glass of Grand Marnier. For a fancier presentation, use two forks to gently pull apart an opening in the middle of each soufflé and drizzle a little Grand Marnier directly into the soufflés. Serve immediately.

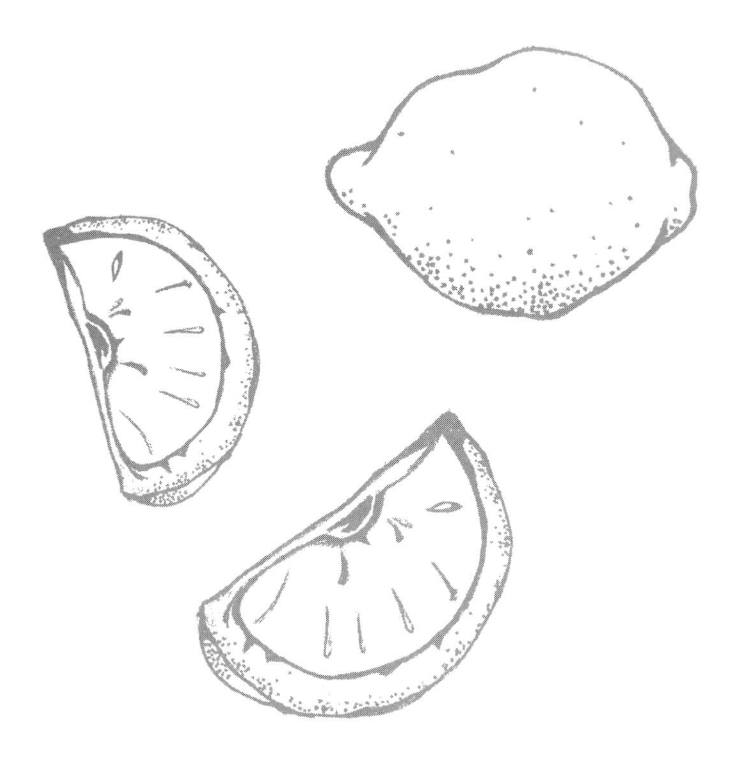

Flourless Chocolate Cake with Fresh Mint Whipped Cream

In Roman times, brides would wear a wreath of mint for luck. You'll be lucky if this scrumptious cake doesn't disappear before you get a piece for yourself!

7 oz semi-sweet chocolate
¾ cup sugar
3 ½ tablespoons butter
1 ½ tablespoons water
½ teaspoon almond extract
5 eggs

1 cup heavy cream
1 tablespoon sugar
1 cup fresh mint leaves

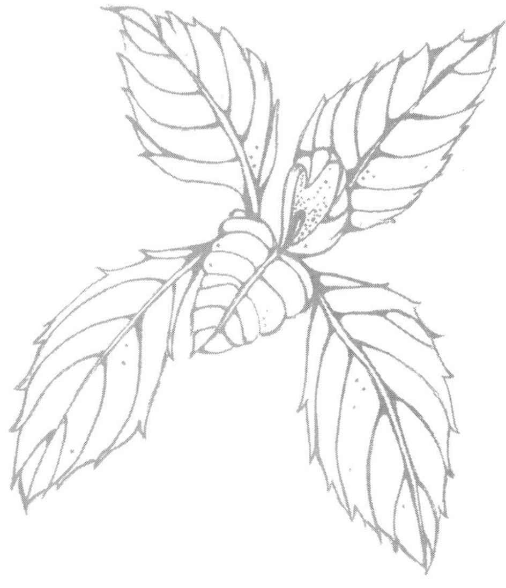

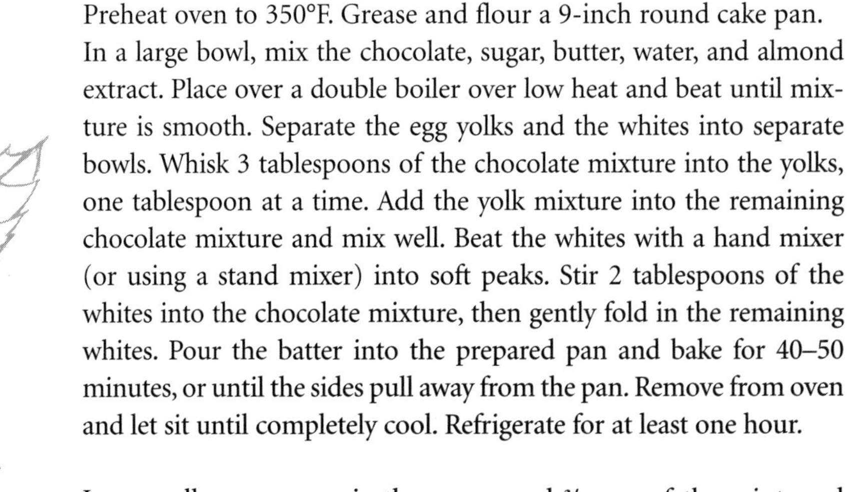

Preheat oven to 350°F. Grease and flour a 9-inch round cake pan. In a large bowl, mix the chocolate, sugar, butter, water, and almond extract. Place over a double boiler over low heat and beat until mixture is smooth. Separate the egg yolks and the whites into separate bowls. Whisk 3 tablespoons of the chocolate mixture into the yolks, one tablespoon at a time. Add the yolk mixture into the remaining chocolate mixture and mix well. Beat the whites with a hand mixer (or using a stand mixer) into soft peaks. Stir 2 tablespoons of the whites into the chocolate mixture, then gently fold in the remaining whites. Pour the batter into the prepared pan and bake for 40–50 minutes, or until the sides pull away from the pan. Remove from oven and let sit until completely cool. Refrigerate for at least one hour.

In a small saucepan, mix the cream and ¾ cup of the mint, and bring to a slow simmer. Cook for 5 minutes. Remove from heat and let steep for a half-hour. Strain through a sieve, pressing on the mint leaves, cover and refrigerate for 1 hour.

When ready to serve, add 1 tablespoon sugar to the cream and whip until firm. Place slices of the cake on serving dishes, dollop with the cream, and garnish with the remaining mint leaves.

Fresh Mint and Citrus Cake

Cake

⅔ cup flour
2 eggs
7 tablespoons salted butter
½ cup sugar
1 tablespoon baking powder
¼ cup fresh lemon juice
1 tablespoon orange zest
1 tablespoon lemon zest
1 tablespoon Grand Marnier
2 tablespoons finely minced mint

Glaze

6 tablespoons fresh orange juice
2 tablespoons Grand Marnier
2 tablespoons butter

It's always fun to throw a barbeque for friends as the days grow warmer, but we sometimes get stuck in the rut of thinking "ice cream" for dessert. Don't get us wrong, we love ice cream, but sometimes it's fun to prepare something a little more unique. This cake is light and refreshing and the aroma of the mint with the citrus is perfect on a summer evening

Preheat oven to 350°F. Beat butter and sugar until creamy. Add eggs and beat until frothy (approximately 1 minute). Add flour and baking powder and stir until completely incorporated. Add mint juice, zests, and Grand Marnier.

Butter and flour a 9 x 5 inch bread loaf pan. Pour in the batter and bake for 50–55 minutes, or until a knife inserted comes out clean. Allow to cool for at least 30 minutes.

Heat glaze ingredients in a small saucepan until dissolved. Prick holes on cakes top with fork. Using a pastry brush, brush the glaze over the cake.

Decorate with fresh mint leaves. Fresh mint whipped cream is delicious with this cake.

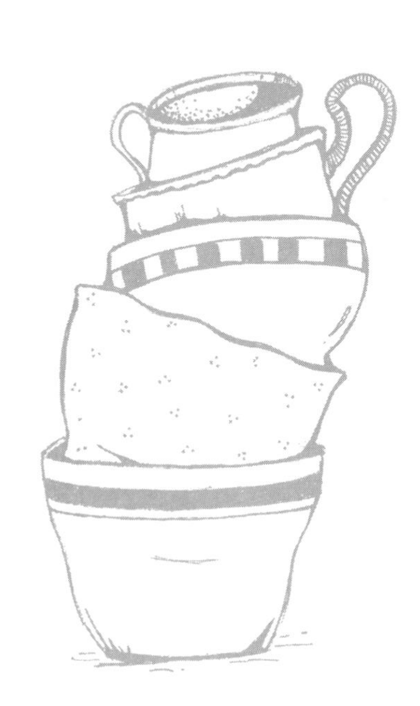

Cardamom Shortbread

Cardamom adds a spicy zip to classic shortbread cookies! These are great to use as a base for our individual fruit "tarts"!

1 stick butter
1 cup flour
¼ cup sugar
⅛ teaspoon salt
½ teaspoon vanilla extract
¼ teaspoon cardamom

Preheat oven to 375°F. In a glass bowl, work all ingredients with your hands to form a soft dough (do not overwork the dough). Press into a shortbread mold, or form into a quarter-inch-thick round or rectangle on a baking sheet. Use a plastic spatula to score the dough into serving pieces. Pierce decoratively with a fork. Bake until just golden, 12–15 minutes. Let cool completely before cutting along the scores.

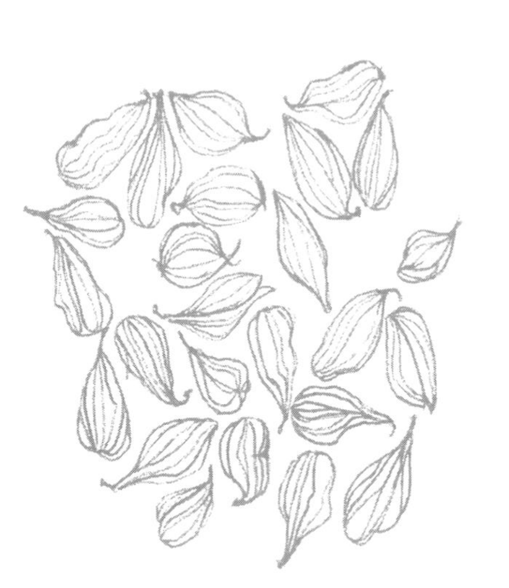

Lemon Verbena Ricotta Pudding

Serves 4–6

¼ cup sugar
1 tablespoon flour
2 eggs and 3egg whites (whites beaten to peaks, yokes set aside)
1 lb fresh ricotta
zest of 1 lemon, finely chopped
2 tablespoons fresh lemon verbena, finely chopped
2 tablespoons orange blossom flower water*

Infused into hot water, lemon verbena creates a wonderfully refreshing tea, which also can aid in digestion.

Preheat oven to 375°F. In a bowl, put ricotta, sugar, flour, orange blossom flower water 2 eggs plus the 3 yokes lemon zest, and lemon verbena. Mix well. Beat the three egg whites to peaks and gently fold into mixture. Pour into a well-greased bundt pan and bake for 35 minutes. Take it out of the oven onto the serving dish of your choice. It is very good served lukewarm.

**Available at specialty food stores*

Minty Fruit Tart

The refreshing aroma and flavor of mint really brighten this beautiful dessert! We like to use raspberries, strawberries, and peaches for their great colors and flavors, but any of your favorite seasonal fruits will work as well!

Shell

1 ¼ cups flour
¼ cup sugar
¼ teaspoon salt
10 tablespoons chilled butter, cut into small pieces
1 egg yolk
3 tablespoons cream
½ teaspoon almond extract

Mint Syrup

½ cup mint leaves
1 cup spring water
⅓ cup sugar

Topping

8 oz mascarpone cheese
⅓ cup mint syrup, above
½ cup raspberries
½ cup strawberries, halved lengthwise
1 peach, sliced

For the Shell

In a food processor, blend the flour, sugar and salt. Add the butter and pulse until the butter is incorporated as a dry blend. Whisk the egg yolk, cream, and almond extract in a small bowl and add to the flour mixture. Process until the dough forms a ball. Press into a flat disk and refrigerate, wrapped in plastic, for 2–4 hours. Preheat oven to 375°F. Press the dough into a tart pan. Cover with aluminum foil and fill with dried beans or pie weights. Bake for about 15 minutes.

Remove foil and beans, and continue baking until shell is golden brown. Remove from oven and let cool.

For the Mint Syrup

In a small saucepan, mix all ingredients and bring to a simmer and cook until syrupy consistency. Strain the syrup, pressing the mint leaves to extract all of the essences. Chill until ready to use.

Blend 1/3 cup of mint syrup into the mascarpone cheese and store covered and chilled until ready to use.

To assemble the tart, spread the mascarpone mixture evenly into the baked and cooled shell. Arrange the fruit decoratively on the tart, saving any extra for another use. Brush the tart with some of the remaining mint syrup. Garnish with a few fresh mint sprigs. Cover with plastic and refrigerate until ready to serve.

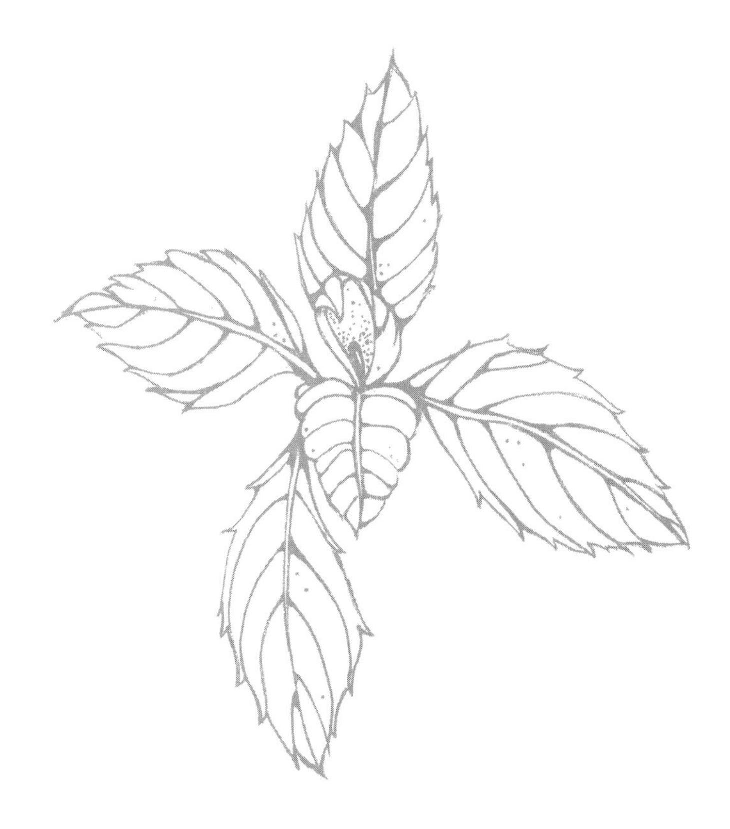

Individual Fruit "Tarts"

This is a quick way to approximate our Minty Fruit Tart if you're pressed for time!

For Each Tart

2 cardamom shortbread cookies (recipe p. 96)
½ cup mixed berries
2 tablespoons Grand Marnier
2 tablespoons crème fraîche (or mascarpone cheese)
2 sprigs of fresh mint

In a glass bowl, pour the liqueur over the berries and let macerate for 15 minutes. Arrange the shortbread in dessert dishes. Dollop with the crème fraîche. Spoon the berries over the cream, and drizzle the dish with the syrup that accumulated in the bottom of the bowl. Garnish with the mint sprigs.

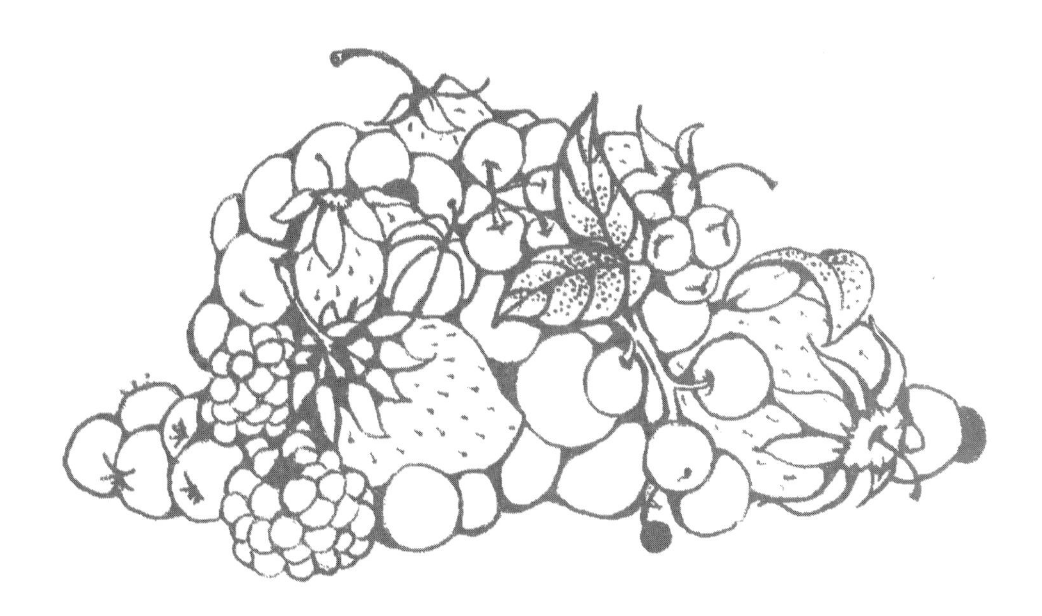

CHAPTER 4

RELAXING BODY, MIND AND SPIRIT:

Recipes that Soothe

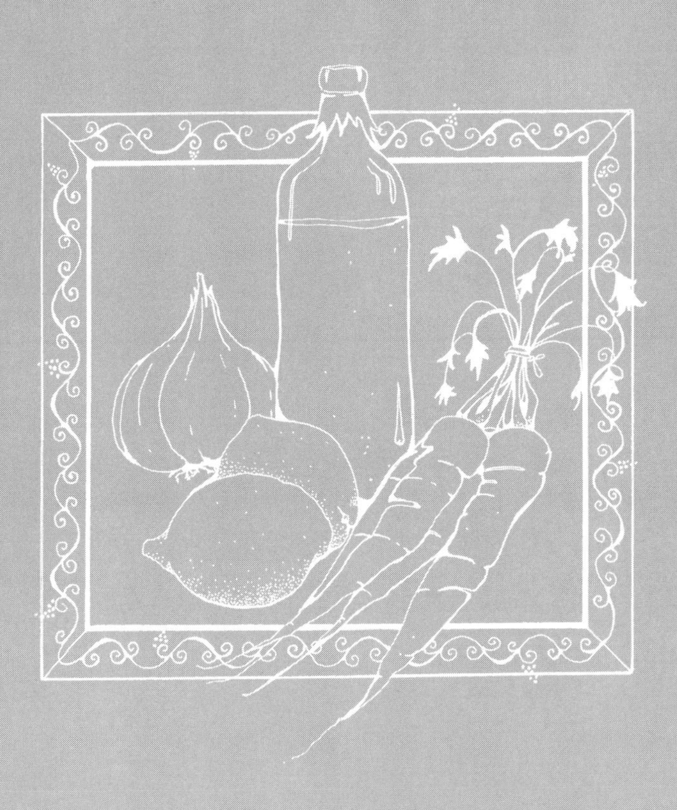

Foods that Soothe

These days it seems like we're always fighting to get things done yesterday. Whether at home or at work, life can be demanding! Sometimes you just have to slow things down, turn off the cell phone and pager, and treat yourself, family and/or friends to a relaxing evening of great food and an atmosphere designed to offer some stress relief through the use of aromatherapy. Proper lighting and color selection are key to creating a perfectly relaxing ambiance (see our chapter on *Creating the Mood*). Of course, the food and its preparation should be soothing as well! In this chapter we offer some great recipes that capitalize on the relaxing properties of commonly available herbs. Put on some comfy clothes, light a candle under some lavender oil, kick back, and flip through the following recipes to find some foods that will fit your soothing mood . . .

Blue Cheese Rösti

Serves 4

Rösti is a classic potato dish from Switzerland—crusty on the outside, soft and creamy inside. In this version, the addition of thyme and blue cheese imparts a warm earthiness that will thrill your palate and soothe the soul.

1½ lb russet potatoes, match-stick cut or shredded
1 tablespoon crushed garlic
2 teaspoons thyme
2 teaspoons chopped parsley
¼ cup crumbled Danish blue cheese
salt and pepper to taste
2 tablespoons olive oil

In a large glass bowl, combine the potatoes with the garlic, thyme, parsley, and salt and pepper and mix well. In a 9-inch nonstick sauté pan, heat 1 tablespoon of the oil over medium-high heat. Press half of the potatoes into the pan. Sprinkle evenly with the blue cheese, and press the remaining potatoes on top, forming an even "pancake." Cover, reduce heat to medium, and cook until a golden brown crust forms on the bottom of the potatoes, and the potatoes are fork-tender. Remove the cover, place a large plate over the potatoes and invert the pan, transferring the potatoes to the plate. Heat the remaining oil in the sauté pan, and slide the potatoes off the plate back into the pan. Cook the potatoes, uncovered, for 5–8 minutes, until the underside has nicely browned and the potatoes are very soft in the center. Serve the potatoes cut into wedges.

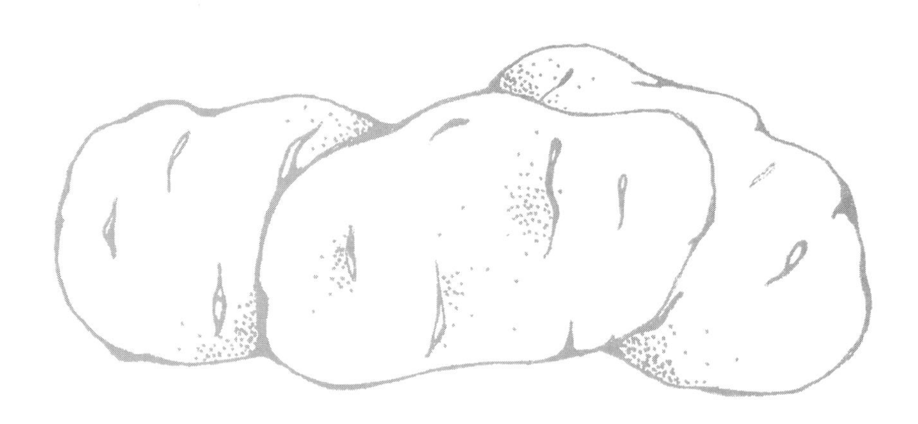

Buckwheat Crêpes with Fresh Basil and Cheese

Serves 4 as a first course or a light entrée

This is a traditional recipe from the coast of Brittany where these crêpes can be bought from vendors on street corners. It is a soothing treat to be enjoyed on a chilly winter day.

Crêpes

2 eggs
1 cup milk
5 tablespoons flour
¼ cup buckwheat flour
½ teaspoon oil
8 teaspoons butter

In a blender, process the eggs, milk, flours, and oil until smooth. Refrigerate for 2 hours. Melt 1 teaspoon butter in a crêpe pan (or a small sauté pan) over medium heat. Use a medium-sized ladle to pour some of the crêpe batter into the pan. Tilt the pan until coated with the batter, and cook until golden, 1–2 minutes per side. Continue with the remaining butter and batter. Transfer the crêpes as they are made to a plate and cover with a moist, clean kitchen towel. Makes 8 crêpes.

Filling

2 tablespoons butter
1 cup milk
8 tablespoons crème fraîche
10 tablespoons finely chopped basil
2 tablespoons flour
freshly grated nutmeg, to taste
½ lb Swiss cheese, grated

In a small saucepan over medium heat, melt the butter. Whisk in the flour until smooth, and cook for 3 minutes. Whisk in the milk, and cook until it just comes to a boil. Season with nutmeg, salt, and pepper; keep warm.

Preheat oven to 350°F. Place 1 tablespoon of fresh basil, 1 tablespoon crème fraîche, and equal amounts of cheese in the center of each crêpe and fold over into a semi-circle. Arrange on a baking sheet, place into oven and bake until the cheese melts, about 5–7 minutes. Divide the crêpes onto four plates, top with sauce and sprinkle with remaining basil. Serve immediately.

Butternut Squash Soup with Sage

Serves 2

> *The word "sage" is derived from the Latin "salvere", meaning "to heal". Sage is well known for its healing properties for mind and body. We certainly find this wonderful autumn soup to be soothing for the soul!*

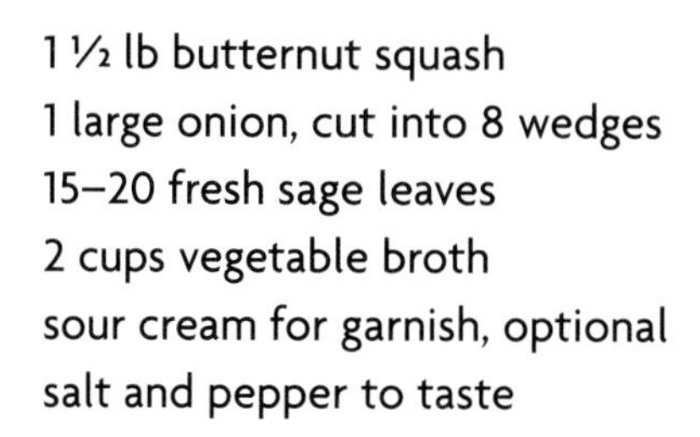

1 ½ lb butternut squash
1 large onion, cut into 8 wedges
15–20 fresh sage leaves
2 cups vegetable broth
sour cream for garnish, optional
salt and pepper to taste

Preheat oven to 375°F. Cut the squash in half lengthwise and remove the seeds. Place cut side down on an oiled baking sheet. Arrange the onion wedges and the whole sage leaves on the baking sheet and roast in the oven for 45 minutes, or until the squash is very soft (check by piercing with a knife at the narrow end, as this is the densest part of the flesh!) Remove from oven and let cool until able to handle. Scoop out the flesh of one squash half into the bowl of a food processor fitted with the steel blade. Add half of the onion, half of the sage, and 1 cup of the broth. Process until very smooth, and transfer to a large saucepan. Process the remaining squash, onion, sage and broth, and add to the saucepan. Heat over medium heat, adjusting the thickness with more broth if desired. Season with salt and pepper. Serve with a dollop of sour cream (or a decorative design from a squeeze bottle), if desired.

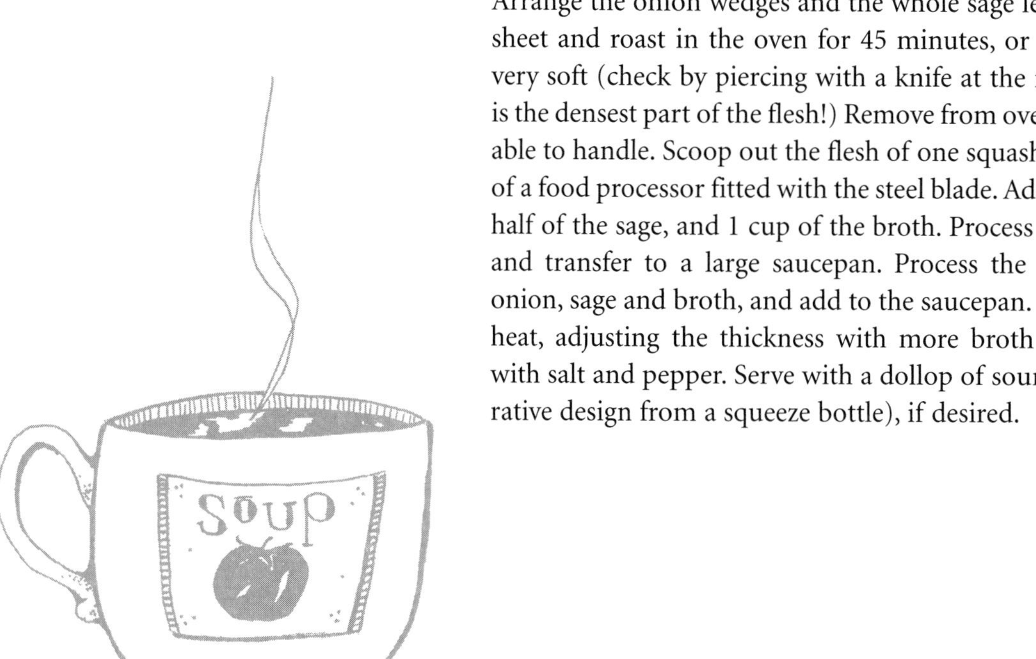

Crab and Thyme Stuffed Mushrooms

Serves 4 as a first course

10 garlic cloves
10 thyme sprigs
1 tablespoon olive oil
6 oz canned crabmeat
6 oz goat cheese, softened
½ teaspoon chopped lemon zest
salt and pepper to taste
12 large mushrooms, stems removed

In ancient Greece, the aroma of thyme was valued as a way to create a sense of elegance and style. This simple and stylish appetizer is sure to please both the palate and the olfactory senses with the tranquil benefits of thyme.

Preheat oven to 400°F. Coat the garlic and thyme sprigs with the oil, and roast in the oven for 25 minutes, until the garlic is softened and golden. In a mixing bowl, pull the thyme leaves from the sprigs and combine with the garlic, crab, goat cheese, lemon zest. Mix until well blended. Season with salt and pepper.

Place the mushrooms on a lightly oiled baking sheet. Mound some of the crab mixture into each mushroom. Bake in the oven until the cheese has just started to melt. Finish under the broiler, if desired, to brown the tops.

Dijon-Lavender Salmon Cakes

Serves 4 as a first course

Ahh, the scent of lavender! It is truly a magical scent, which conjures tranquil and healing benefits to the soul. Its amazing aroma will blanket your kitchen with serenity as you prepare these delicious little salmon cakes.

1 tablespoon olive oil
1 large shallot, minced
2 teaspoons dried lavender
2 6-oz cans boneless, skinless salmon
1 teaspoon grated lemon zest
1 teaspoon fresh lemon juice
1 ½ tablespoons Dijon mustard
⅓ cup dried breadcrumbs
1 egg

mixed baby greens and balsamic vinaigrette, for serving

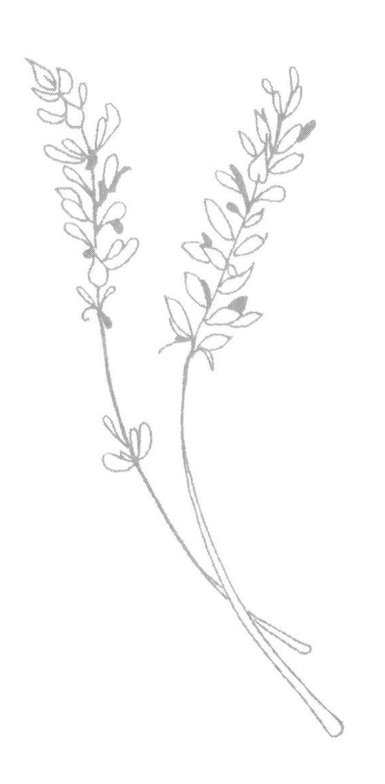

In a small skillet, heat the oil over high heat and sauté the shallot for 3 minutes. Add the lavender and quickly sauté, until the lavender aroma is released. Remove from heat and let cool.

Flake the salmon into a mixing bowl. Add the lemon zest, lemon juice, mustard, breadcrumbs, egg, and the cooled shallot/lavender mixture. Combine with a fork until well blended. Form the mixture into eight small cakes, and place on a plate lined with waxed paper. Cover with another sheet of waxed paper and refrigerate for 30 minutes.

Heat a non-stick skillet over medium heat. Cook the salmon cakes until they are nicely browned on both sides, about 5 minutes per side. To serve, toss the greens with some vinaigrette and place onto four small plates. Place two crab cakes on each plate and drizzle the cakes with a little more vinaigrette.

Chamomile Quiche

Serves 4–6

2 cups milk
¼ cup chamomile flowers (dried)
½ tablespoon chamomile oil (can substitute canola)
1 leek, diced
3 eggs
1 cup grated Monterey Jack cheese

9-inch prepared pie crust

The soothing nature of chamomile makes this a natural for a relaxing Sunday brunch. Well, a little champagne might help, too!

In a small saucepan, combine the milk and the chamomile. Bring to a simmer over low heat, being careful not to burn the milk. Remove from heat, cover, and allow to steep for 20 minutes. Strain through a sieve into a measuring cup.

Meanwhile, heat the oil in a skillet over medium-high heat. Sauté the leek until very soft, 10 minutes. Remove from heat.

Preheat oven to 375°F. Whisk the eggs in a medium mixing bowl. Slowly whisk in the milk until fully incorporated. Spread the leeks into the bottom of the pie crust, sprinkle evenly with the cheese, and slowly cover with the egg mixture. Place on a baking sheet and bake for 25–30 minutes, or until the custard has set.

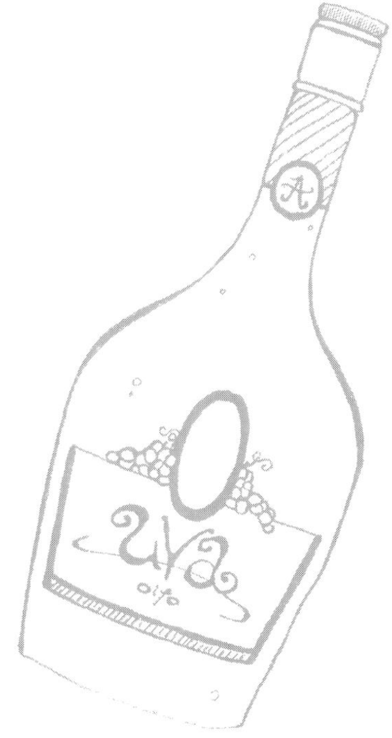

Sage and Potato Frittata

Serves 2

Eggs need not be relegated to simply breakfast foods—sometimes it's good to think out of the box (or in this case, the egg carton)! The earthiness of sage comforts the senses and makes this a natural for an informal supper on a crisp autumn evening.

4 tablespoons canola oil
1 cup sliced onions
1 cup peeled, diced potatoes
3 tablespoons minced fresh sage
1 cup diced tomato
6 eggs, beaten
½ cup crumbled Feta cheese
salt and pepper to taste

Preheat oven to 350°F. In an oven proof 12-inch skillet, heat the oil over medium heat. Add the onions and potatoes and sauté for 8–10 minutes. Add the tomatoes and cook for another 4–5 minutes. Sprinkle the sage over the vegetables. Pour the eggs over the vegetables and cook, lifting the eggs as they start to cook so that the uncooked portion will run under the cooked portion. When the eggs are starting to set, but are still runny, place the pan in the oven and cook for 3–5 minutes, or until the eggs are set. Remove from the oven and sprinkle with the feta cheese. Cut into serving wedges.

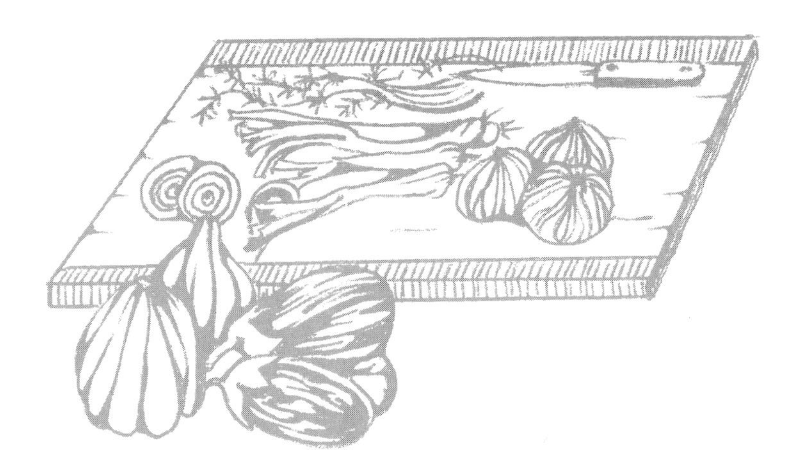

Mesclun Salad with Warm Thyme Vinaigrette

Serves 4

¼ cup olive oil
½ oz wild mushrooms, fresh or dried
3 shallots, cut into 1/4 inch wedges
¼ cup chopped red bell pepper
½ tablespoon thyme
1 ½ tablespoons red wine vinegar
¼ cup Pinot Noir, or other dry red wine
3 oz mesclun (mixed baby greens)
3 tablespoons chopped walnuts*
salt and pepper to taste

This salad pairs perfectly with Goat Cheese Soufflés with Roasted Garlic and Thyme. Toss in the warm vinaigrette just before serving.

If using dried mushrooms, reconstitute in ½ cup of warm water for 20 minutes. Drain, then chop. In a small sauté pan, heat the olive oil over medium heat. Add the mushrooms, shallot, red bell pepper, thyme and sauté for 5 minutes. Add the vinegar and continue cooking for 3 minutes. Add the wine and cook until the vegetables are very soft and the wine is reduced by about half. Salt and pepper to taste. Remove from heat. Place the mesclun into a wood salad bowl. Toss with the vinaigrette and sprinkle with the walnuts.

**If desired, use candied walnuts, available in the produce section of most markets.*

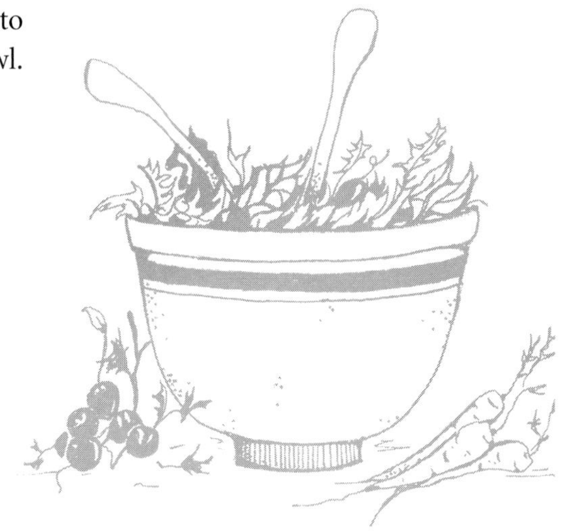

Roasted Vegetables with Thyme Vinaigrette

Serves 4

This recipe makes a superb accompaniment to grilled chicken or fish, but we have also found that it works very well tossed with pasta and topped with shaved parmesan.

½ cup olive oil
2 tablespoons balsamic vinegar
4 tablespoons chopped fresh thyme
salt and pepper

3 potatoes
6 beets
6 carrots
3 red onions
12 garlic cloves (unpeeled)

Preheat oven to 400°F.
Cut all vegetables into 1-inch pieces. In a large bowl, whisk together the vinaigrette ingredients. Add the vegetables and toss until well coated. Spread the mixture onto a large baking sheet and bake for 1 hour, stirring occasionally.

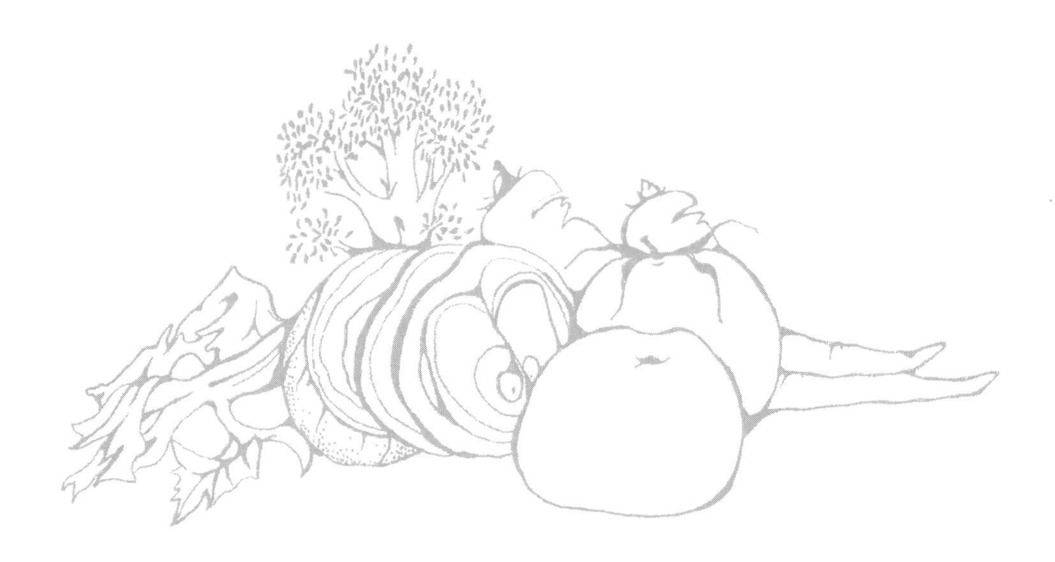

Grilled Chicken with Sage Cream Sauce

Serves 4–6

6 boneless, skinless chicken breasts
½ cup olive oil
½ cup fresh lemon juice
3 garlic cloves, minced
salt and pepper

2 cups heavy cream
1 cup finely chopped sage
1 garlic clove, finely chopped
1 teaspoon fresh lemon juice

Sage is an herb that has long been associated with a sense of well-being, and for good reason! Sage accentuates mental clarity, aids in digestion, and assuages aches and pains. There is an old tradition of hanging sprigs of sage in a window when a loved one sets out on a journey—if the sage stays fresh you can be assured that your loved one is well!

In a flat dish, mix the olive oil, lemon juice, garlic, and salt and pepper to taste. Add the chicken and marinate, turning once, for 4 hours, or overnight. Grill the chicken over hot coals until just cooked, about 6 minutes per side. (Alternately, the chicken can be cooked under a heated broiler.)

While the chicken is cooking, make the sauce. Put the cream in a medium saucepan and reduce at a rolling boil over medium heat for 10 minutes, or until reduced by half. Add the sage, garlic, lemon, and salt and pepper to taste. Cook for 5 minutes. Remove from heat and let stand for 5 minutes. Pour the mixture into a blender (or use a hand-held mixer) and process until thoroughly blended.

Place the chicken over cooked rice or couscous, and drape with the sauce. Garnish with a few whole sage leaves.

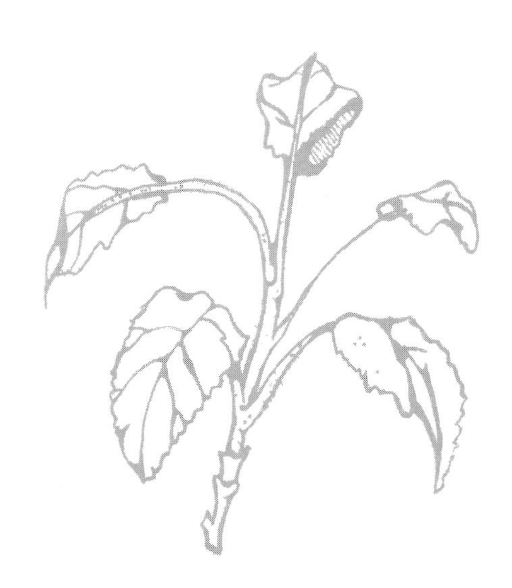

Lavender Lasagna

Serves 8

Admittedly, this lasagna takes some time to prepare, but it's well worth the effort! The aroma from the lavender is intoxicating and soothing. It's hard to describe just how luscious this is, and how calming the aromas! You'll just have to try it for yourself and see! It's a perfect dish to make for a relaxing evening with family and friends.

1 stick butter (½ cup)
½ cup flour
4 cups milk
1 ½ cups freshly grated parmesan

2 large eggplants (1 ½ lb each)
2 tablespoons olive oil
1 onion, chopped
5 garlic cloves, sliced
2 large portabello mushrooms, cut into 1 inch pieces
1 red bell pepper, cut into 1-inch pieces
2 tablespoons dried lavender flowers
2 cups dry red wine
3 medium tomatoes, chopped (use a 14-oz can if fresh not available)

1 lb lasagna noodles
1 cup Gruyere cheese

Preheat oven to 375°F. In a saucepan, melt the butter over medium heat. Add the flour, stir until thoroughly incorporated, and cook for 3 minutes, stirring constantly. Add the milk, and continue stirring until the liquid just comes to a boil, about 10 minutes. Stir in ½ cup of the parmesan cheese. Cover and set aside.

Prick the eggplants with a fork and roast in the oven for 20–30 minutes, or until very soft. Remove from oven and let cool.

In a large skillet with raised sides (or a large saucepan), heat the oil over medium-high heat. Add the onion and sauté until just translucent, about 3 minutes. Add the garlic, mushrooms, and bell pepper, season with salt and pepper and cook another 3 minutes. Add the lavender and cook for 5 minutes. Cut the eggplants in half and scoop the flesh into the pot with a large spoon, breaking up the flesh. Pour in the wine and tomatoes. Cook over medium-high heat, stirring occasionally, for 20 minutes. Season with salt and pepper.

While the veggies are cooking, bring a large pot of salted water to a boil and cook the lasagne noodles until just al dente. Drain into a colander and rinse under cold water. Let the noodles drain until nearly dry, or pat with a paper towel to remove excess water.

To assemble the lasagna, spread about half-cup of the veggie mixture onto the bottom of a 9 x 12 lasagna pan. Cover by overlapping 4 lasagna noodles. Spoon another portion of the veggie mixture over the noodles, then drop several tablespoons of the cream sauce over the vegetables and smooth it with the back of a spoon. Sprinkle with some of the remaining parmesan. Continue layering with noodles, veggies, sauce and cheese, finishing with a top layer of noodles and cream sauce. Sprinkle the rest of the parmesan and the Gruyere over the top and bake for 30–40 minutes, or until the top is golden and the lasagna is bubbling. Remove from oven and let rest for 10 minutes before cutting and serving.

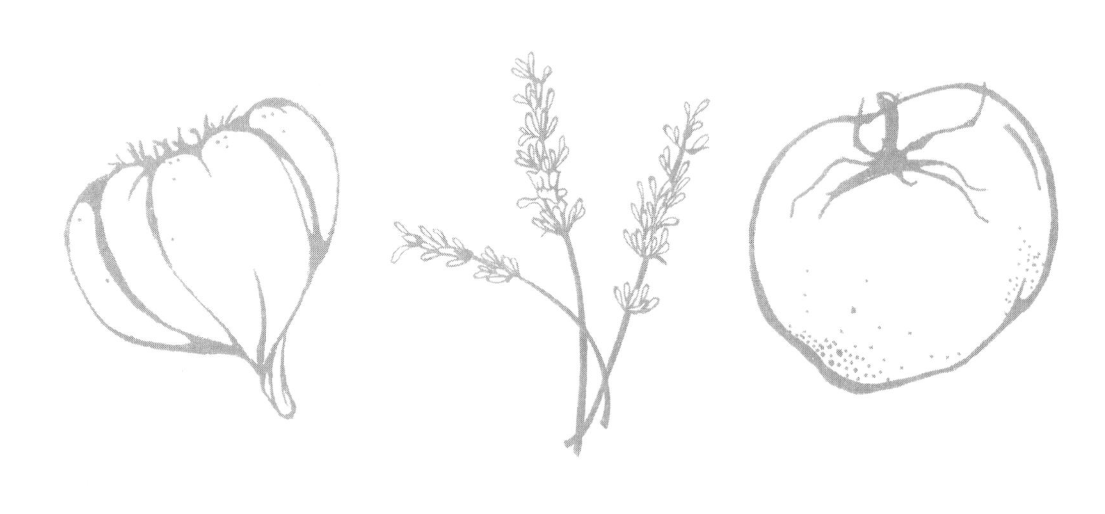

Oregano Chicken with Polenta and Feta

Serves 4

Oregano is an herb of happiness and comfort. This dish will serve you well in making dinner guests happy, as it not only tastes great but makes for a stunning presentation.

Polenta

1 cup corn meal
1 ½ cups chicken broth
1 ½ cups milk
salt and pepper to taste

Chicken

4 boneless, skinless chicken breast halves
½ cup chopped oregano
4 garlic cloves, crushed
juice of 1 lemon
2 tablespoons olive oil
freshly ground pepper

Garnish

3 medium tomatoes, seeded and chopped
½ tablespoon balsamic vinegar
1 tablespoon olive oil
6 oz crumbled feta cheese

Make the polenta one day ahead. In a large saucepan, bring the chicken broth and milk to a simmer. Slowly whisk in the corn meal and cook, stirring frequently, for 20 minutes. Add salt and pepper to taste. Pour the polenta into an 8-inch square pan and smooth with a spatula. Cover and refrigerate overnight.

Reserve about 2 tablespoons of oregano for garnish. Mix the remaining oregano with the garlic, lemon, olive oil, and pepper to taste. Coat the chicken breasts with the herb mixture, and refrigerate for 20 minutes. Heat a nonstick skillet with a small amount of oil over medium-high heat. Add the chicken and brown on both sides, creating an herb "crust." Lower the heat to medium and continue cooking until the chicken is just cooked, about 15 minutes.

Meanwhile, remove the polenta from the refrigerator and cut into 8 triangle-shaped pieces. Heat a ridged grill pan over medium-high heat. Brush the triangles with olive oil and add to the pan, cooking for about 5–7 minutes on each side, or until colored with grill marks.

To serve, place 2 pieces of polenta in each of four large shallow bowls, with triangle points meeting in the center. Toss the tomatoes with the vinegar and oil, and spoon decoratively across the points and around the polenta. Drape one piece of chicken over the polenta in each bowl, sprinkle with the feta and reserved oregano.

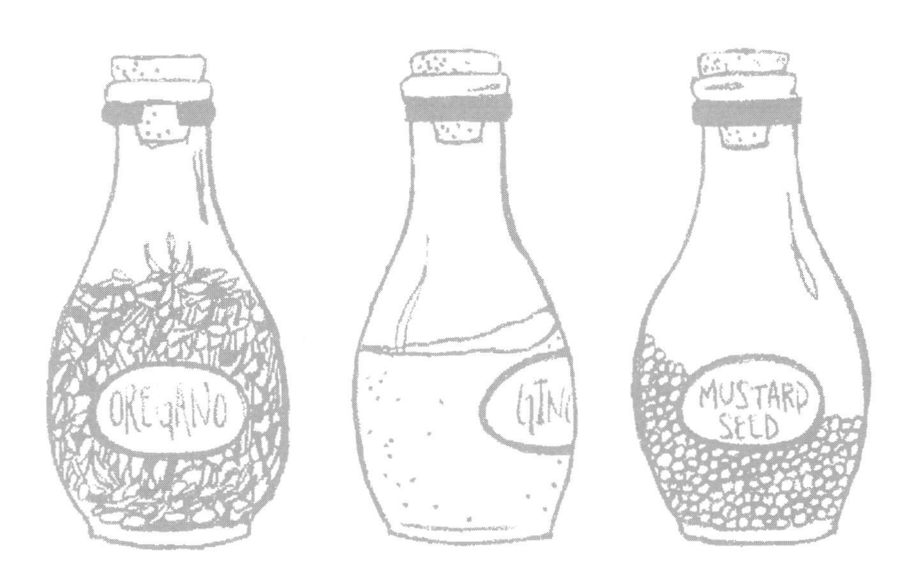

Tomato Linguine a la Chamomile Checca

Serves 2

The addition of chamomile in this twist on the classic pasta a la checca might strike you as a bit strange—it did us—but we tried it anyway and found it fabulous! As always, working with chamomile is soothing to the soul.

8 oz homemade-style tomato linguine

½ cup chamomile oil
6 shallots, sliced into wedges
6 plum tomatoes, seeded and diced
1 cup sliced mushrooms
salt and pepper

½ cup minced fresh basil

Cook the pasta in a large pot of salted boiling water until just al dente. Drain and rinse with warm water. Wipe out the pot with a paper towel and return to the stove. Heat the chamomile oil over medium heat, and cook the shallots until softened, about 5 minutes. Add the tomato and mushrooms, season with salt and pepper, and cook for 2-3 minutes. Return the pasta to the pot and stir until coated with the oil and heated through. Divide the pasta into serving bowls and sprinkle with the basil.

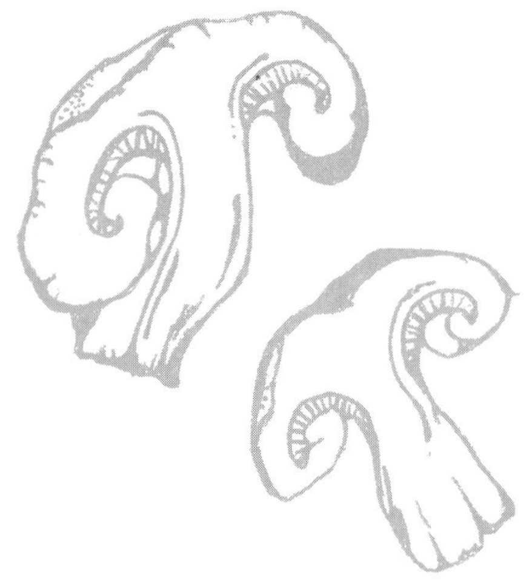

Red Wine and Sage Risotto with Wild Mushrooms

Serves 4

1 oz dried mixed wild mushrooms
1 cup hot water
1 ½ cups vegetable stock
1 cup dry red wine
1 tablespoon olive oil
1 large shallot, chopped
1 cup Arborio rice
¼ cup minced fresh sage
salt and pepper to taste
shaved parmesan cheese, for garnish

Sage is lauded for relieving feelings of grief and anxiety. This combination of red wine, sage, and wild mushrooms works wonders in creating an earthy sense of contentment.

In a small bowl, cover the mushrooms with the hot water and let sit for 15 minutes. Drain the liquid into a medium saucepan, and roughly chop the mushrooms. Add the stock and wine to the saucepan and bring to a low simmer. In another saucepan, heat the oil over medium-high heat. Sauté the shallot until translucent. Add the rice and sage, and stir until well coated. Cook for 3 minutes. Add the mushrooms and sauté for another 2–3 minutes. Season with salt and pepper. With a ladle, begin adding the liquid to the rice, one ladle at a time, stirring until nearly all of the liquid is absorbed before adding the next ladle. Continue adding the liquid in this manner until the rice is just al dente, and the sauce is velvety and thickened. Re-season with salt and pepper to taste and serve immediately, garnished with shaved parmesan.

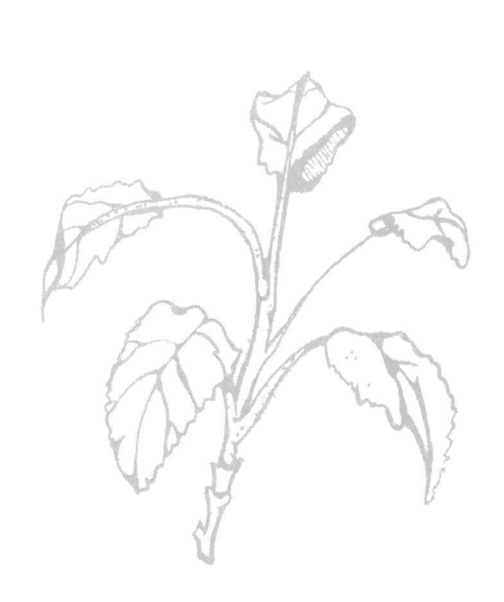

Eggplant and Basil Gratin

Serves 4–6

This is an outstanding and warming dish to serve either as a main course or a side dish. It will serve 4 as an entrée, or 6 as a side dish. The basil not only imparts its wonderful flavor and aroma, but is also well known to aid in digestion—just the ticket for creating a soothing mood! A simple salad of arugula with shaved parmesan makes a great accompaniment to the gratin.

½ cup olive oil
1 onion, diced
2 large eggplants, diced
2 potatoes, boiled, peeled, and diced
2 tablespoons salt
1 tablespoon pepper
1 lb tomatoes, diced
1 tablespoon thyme
1 cup basil, minced
16 oz fresh mozzarella, sliced

2 tablespoons olive oil

Preheat oven to 350°F. In a large skillet heat ½ cup oil over medium heat. Add the onion, eggplant, potatoes, and salt and pepper and sauté for 10–12 minutes, or until eggplant is tender. Add the tomatoes and thyme and cook for another 5 minutes.

Oil the bottom and sides of a large baking dish with the remaining 2 tablespoons olive oil. Layer ¼ of the eggplant mixture into the dish, and cover with ½ cup basil and half of the mozzarella. Repeat with another layer of eggplant, basil, and cheese. Bake for 18–20 minutes, or until the mozzarella is bubbly and golden.

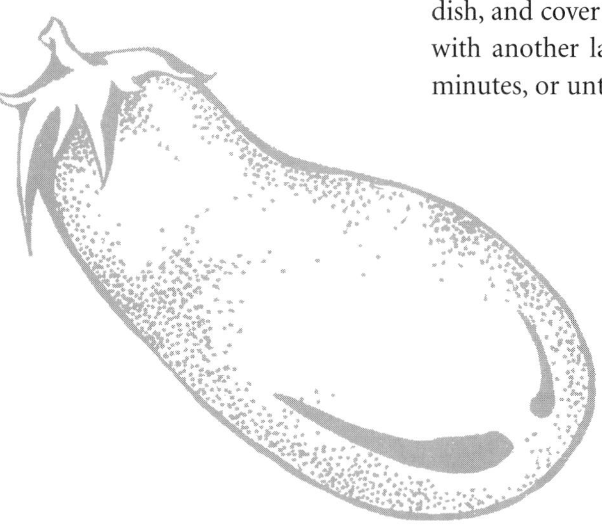

Sage Stuffed Tomatoes

Serves 6–8

8–10 medium tomatoes
2 slices white bread
½ cup milk
1 ½ lb ground turkey
12 oz bulk pork sausage
2–2 ½ cups cooked rice
1 egg
½ cup minced sage
2 garlic cloves, minced
1 tablespoon cracked pepper
2 scallions, sliced
1 cup Swiss cheese

Since ancient times, sage has been attributed with not only longevity, but also immortality! The Latin phrase "cur moriatur homo cui salvia crescit in horto?" translates to "why should a man die whilst sage grows in his garden?"

Preheat oven to 400°F. Cut a round in the top of the tomatoes and scoop out the seeds to make hollow shells. Let drain inverted on paper towels.

In a large mixing bowl, soak the bread in the milk until all of the liquid has been absorbed. Add the next eight ingredients to the bowl and mix well with your hands. (Remember, good cooking is about using *all* of your five senses!) Fill the tomatoes with the stuffing and place in a lightly oiled shallow-sided baking dish. Bake the tomatoes for 40 minutes, top with the cheese and bake an additional 6–8 minutes, or until melted and browned.

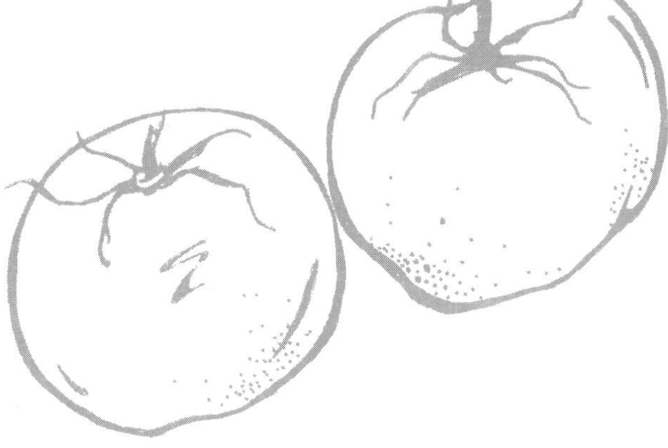

Herb-Crusted Halibut with Creamy Polenta

Serves 4

Great textures and flavors play off of each other wonderfully to create a satisfying and relaxing dish. Try pairing it with some pan grilled vegetables to round out the meal. Don't worry about leftovers—there won't be any!

Herb Mix

2 tablespoons minced oregano
2 tablespoons minced basil
1 tablespoon minced thyme

Halibut

4 halibut steaks, about ½ lb each
¼ cup herb mix
¼ teaspoon cayenne pepper
½ cup dried breadcrumbs
salt and pepper to taste
¼ cup mayonnaise
2 teaspoons olive oil

Polenta

1 ½ cups chicken or vegetable broth
2 ½ cups milk
1 cup yellow corn meal
2 tablespoons chopped sundried tomatoes (packed in oil, drained)
½ cup grated parmesan
1 tablespoon herb mix

Start the polenta. In a 2-qt saucepan, combine the broth and the milk and bring to a simmer. Stream in the cornmeal, whisking until smooth. Cook the polenta over low heat, not bringing above a simmer, for 40 minutes stirring frequently. Stir in the sundried tomatoes, parmesan, and herbs. Cover and keep over low heat until ready to serve.

While the polenta is cooking, combine 1/4 cup of the herb mix with the breadcrumbs, cayenne, and salt and pepper to taste in a shallow dish. Heat the olive oil in a medium skillet over medium-high heat. Coat one side of the fish with a thin layer of mayonnaise. Press into the herb mixture, spread the other side with mayonnaise and flip the fish to coat the other side. Transfer to the skillet. Repeat with remaining fish pieces. Reduce heat to medium and cook until the underside is evenly browned, about 5 minutes. Carefully turn the fish and continue cooking for another 5 minutes or until the fish is just opaque.

To serve, spoon a portion of the polenta onto each of four plates, and place a piece of fish such that half of it rests on the bed of polenta.

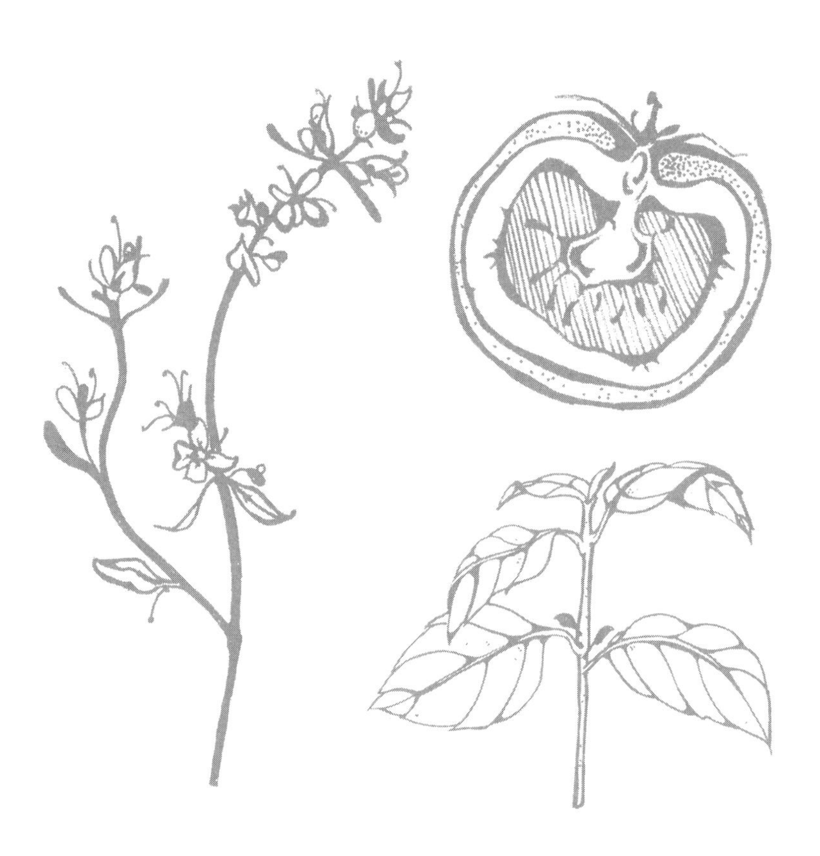

Herb Roasted Artichokes

Serves 4

The aroma of thyme relieves stress and is an herbal way to treat melancholy and nightmares! These fabulous artichokes look great and will go far to inspire happy dreams!

2 large artichokes
3 tablespoons minced thyme
3 tablespoons minced oregano
½ cup balsamic vinegar
½ cup olive oil

Trim the artichoke stems, leaving about 1 inch of stem. Steam the artichokes for 45 minutes. Cut in half lengthwise and remove the choke.

Preheat oven to 500°F. Whisk together the thyme, oregano, vinegar, and oil. Place the artichoke halves in a baking dish and drizzle with the vinaigrette. Roast in the oven for 15 minutes, or until the outer leaves start to blacken. Serve with some homemade mayonnaise, if desired, but we think the vinaigrette is flavoring enough!

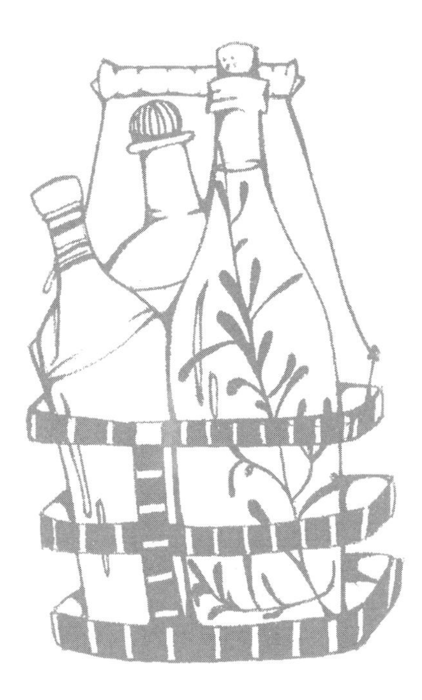

Pan-Grilled Vegetables

Serves 2

2 small zucchini
2 medium carrots
2 Japanese eggplants
1 tablespoon minced sage
1 tablespoon mince thyme
1 tablespoon minced rosemary
1 garlic clove, minced
½ tablespoon freshly ground black pepper
¼ cup olive oil

Crisp grilled vegetables studded with savory herbs complement most any meal! Though great prepared over a charcoal grill, it's easy to do in the kitchen at any time of year with the aid of a ridged grill pan.

Trim and slice each of the vegetables lengthwise into ¼-inch slices. Whisk the herbs, garlic, and pepper with the olive oil. Place the veggies in a shallow dish, and drizzle with the herb mixture. Heat a ridged grill pan over medium-high to high heat. Place the veggies in a single layer in the pan and cook, turning once, until just softened and nicely marked on both sides.

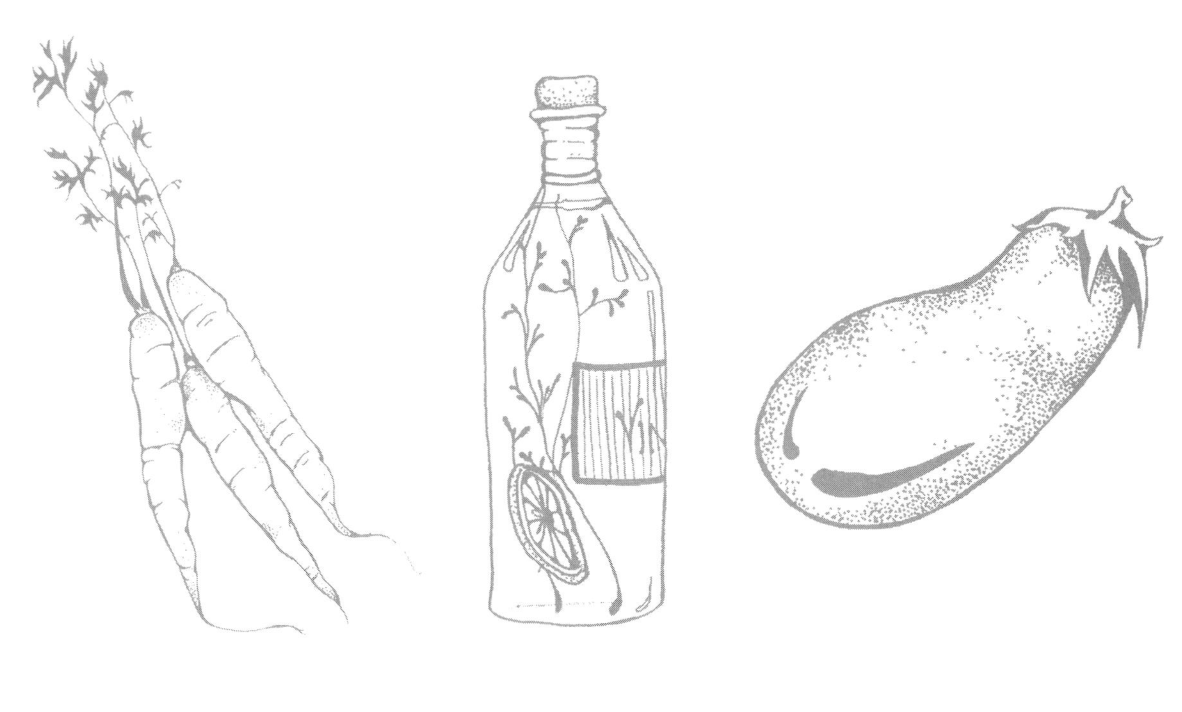

Goat Cheese Soufflés with Roasted Garlic and Thyme

Serves 2

The scent of thyme inspires a relaxed mood, and is a classic herb to pair with goat cheese. Take your time preparing this recipe and enjoy the soothing benefits!

1 head garlic, whole
1 tablespoon olive oil
3 tablespoons butter
3 tablespoons flour
1 cup milk
4 eggs, separated
8 oz goat cheese
1 tablespoon thyme
butter for preparing ramekins

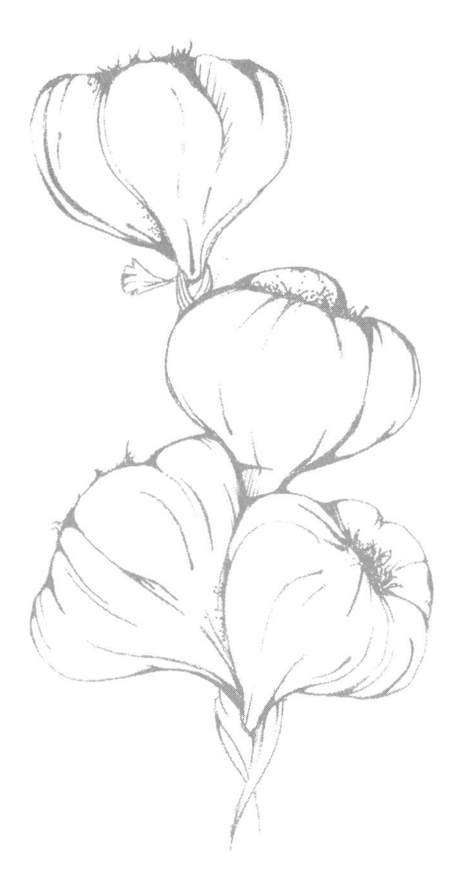

Preheat oven to 400°F. Cut the top off of the head of garlic, place on a piece of aluminum foil, and drizzle with the olive oil. Roast for 30–40 minutes, until very soft and browned.

Reduce the oven heat to 375°F. In a saucepan, melt the butter over medium heat. Add the flour and cook, stirring, for 3 minutes. Add the milk and cook until the milk just comes to a boil, stirring constantly. Remove from heat. Squeeze the garlic cloves from the head directly into the sauce. Add the egg yolks, goat cheese, and thyme and blend thoroughly. Can be prepared a couple of hours in advance—store covered.

Place the egg whites in the bowl of a stand mixer. Beat with the whisk attachment until they form soft peaks (the tip of the peak should just curl over when the whisk is lifted from the whites). Stir 1/4 of the whites into the sauce base. Transfer the sauce base to the bowl with the remaining whites and fold gently to incorporate. Pour the soufflé mix into two 2-cup buttered ramekins. Place the ramekins into a baking dish and add simmering water to come half way up the sides of the ramekins. Place in the oven and bake for 25 minutes, or until nicely puffed and browned. Serve immediately.

Sage-Zucchini Pancakes with Tomato-Mint Coulis

Serves 2

4 tablespoons olive oil
2 zucchini, diced
2 garlic cloves, crushed
¼ cup chopped onion
¾ cup flour
1 tablespoon baking powder
¼ cup parmesan
1 tablespoon minced sage
½ cup milk
salt and pepper

3 medium tomatoes
¼ cup mint, minced (plus whole leaves for garnish)
1 tablespoon olive oil
salt and pepper

An old English proverb states that "He that would live for aye, Must eat sage in May", harkening to the healthful benefits of sage. As zucchini is abundant in the spring, this is a great way to embody the proverb!

For the Pancakes
Sauté the zucchini with the onion and garlic in 2 tablespoons of olive oil for 5 minutes. In a bowl, mix together the flour, baking powder, parmesan, and sage. Stir in the milk. Add the sautéed vegetables and mix. Heat the remaining 2 tablespoons oil in a skillet and add the batter to make pancakes. Cook 3–4 minutes per side, or until browned.

For the Coulis
Parboil the tomatoes for 45 seconds, then plunge into ice water. Remove the skin. Dice the tomatoes, removing all seeds. Puree with a hand mixer until smooth. Add the mint, oil, and salt and pepper to taste. Serve with the pancakes, garnishing with fresh mint leaves.

Chamomile Risotto

Serves 2–4

> *Chamomile was often used as a bed for garden walkways, releasing its comforting powers with each step. Amazingly, it actually thrived instead of withering with foot traffic, which led to an old saying—"Like a chamomile bed, the more it is trodden, the more it will spread."*

¼ cup chamomile flowers, dried
1 ½ cups white wine
1 cup chicken broth
1 shallot, minced
1 cup arborio rice
olive oil
salt and pepper

In a saucepan, combine the chamomile, wine, and broth. Bring to a simmer and let seep for 20 minutes. Strain through a sieve into a bowl. Keep warm. In another saucepan, sauté the shallot in a small amount of olive oil until softened, about 2 minutes. Add the rice and stir until the rice is coated with the oil, and continue to sauté for 5 minutes. Add ½ cup of the liquid to the rice and stir constantly until absorbed. Continue to add the liquid in ½–⅓ cup portions, stirring constantly, until the mixture has a creamy consistency and the rice is tender to the bite. Season with salt and pepper, and serve immediately. (*Note:* you may not use all of the liquid, depending on the particular rice and the heat under the pan.)

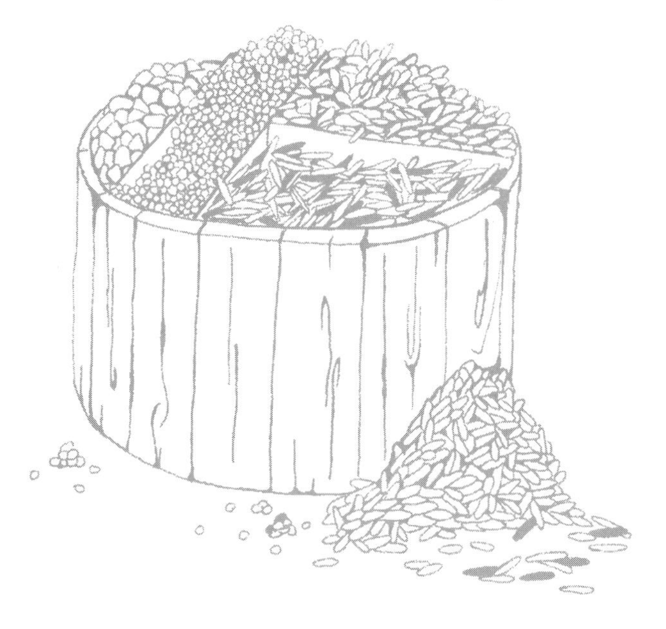

Chamomile Crème Caramel

2 ¼ cups sugar
¼ cup water
5–6 drops lemon juice
3 ¼ cups milk
1 cup dried chamomile flowers
4 whole eggs, plus 3 egg yolks

Sensuous crème caramel with the addition of relaxing chamomile makes this a perfect and elegant ending to any meal.

Preheat oven to 325°F. In a 9-inch round cake pan, combine 1½ cups of the sugar with the water and lemon juice. Heat stirring until the sugar is dissolved, the bring to a boil over high heat for 8–10 minutes. *Do not overcook!* The caramel syrup should be a rich golden brown, but any darker will cause bitterness.

Combine the milk and chamomile in a medium saucepan. Bring to a low boil. Remove from heat, cover, and allow to steep for 20–30 minutes.

In a bowl, mix the eggs, egg yolks and remaining sugar. Slowly strain the milk through a sieve into the egg mixture, whisking constantly so as not to cook the eggs. Place the cake pan with the caramel into a large roasting pan. Pour the custard over the caramel, and add one inch of simmering water to the bottom of the roasting pan to ensure even cooking. Bake for 40–50 minutes, or until the custard is firm to the touch. Chill for at least 4 hours before serving.

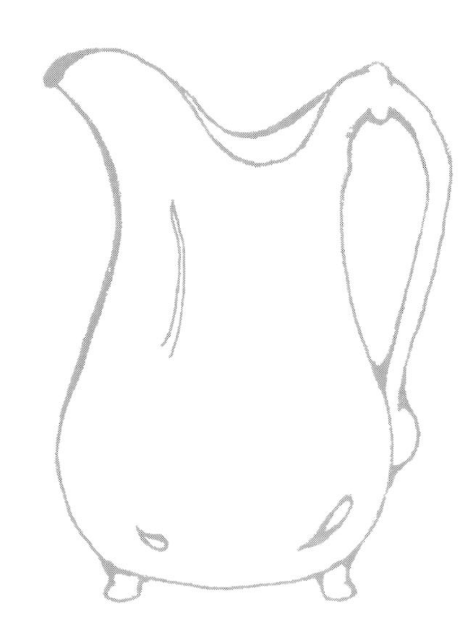

CHAPTER 5

HEALING YOUR INNER CHILD: Recipes that Comfort

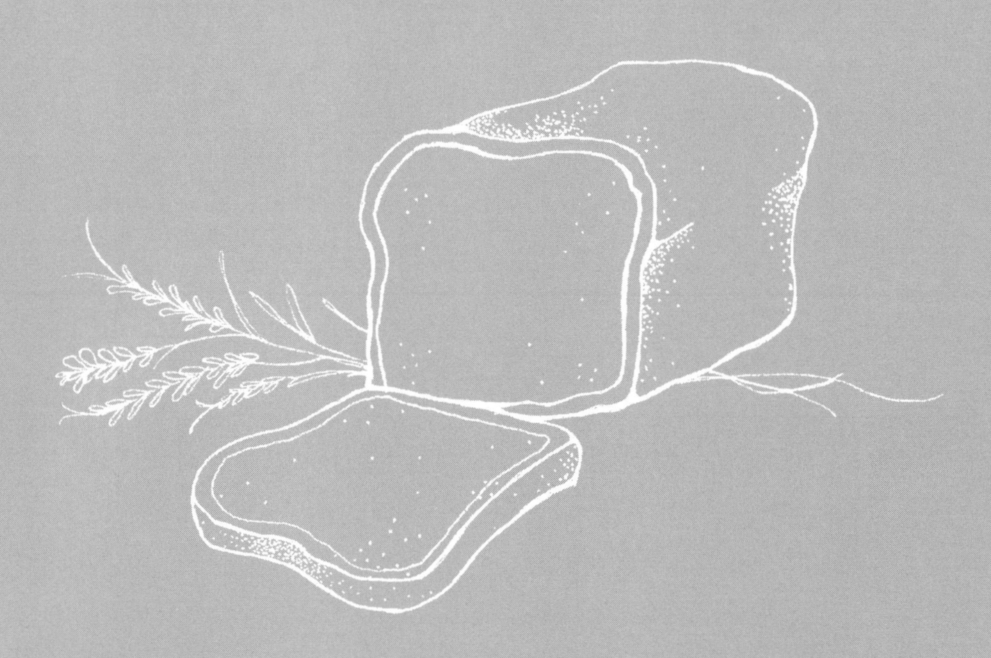

Comfort Food

The concept of "comfort food" is naturally subjective. Instead of relying on the chemical and clinical properties of herbs and flowers, we simply give over to the aromatic sense memories that are conjured up when the smell of freshly baking bread is in the air, or when we recreate a classic dish from our childhood. People's ideas of what constitutes a comfort food can vary widely, often depending on the geographical region in which they grew up and the foods and herbs that are abundant in those areas. We asked several of our friends from all over the world to share with us a favorite comfort food. Here, in their own writing, are their picks, along with a few of our own! We hope that the aromas that they emanate will penetrate your soul with the comfort of a loving hug! Perhaps you will adopt at least one or two into your own anthology of "comfort foods."

Meatloaf

Serves 6

What comfort food chapter would be complete without meatloaf? Although it may have a reputation as rather pedantic, it is always near the top of everyone's favorites list! Serve this classic with garlic mashed potatoes and you will receive rave reviews!

⅓ red onion minced
1 lb ground turkey
1 lb bulk turkey or pork sausage
½ cup shredded Parmesan cheese
3 tablespoons no-fat sour cream
¼ teaspoon garlic powder
⅛ teaspoon black pepper
5 tablespoons julienned fresh basil
2 teaspoons Dijon mustard
14 ½ oz chopped can of tomatoes with juice
2 egg bagels, processed into crumbs
1 large egg

Preheat oven to 350°F. Mix all ingredients together in a large bowl (except about 2 tablespoons of the Parmesan cheese) with your hands (clean of course). This is really the only way to mix this properly! Press the mixture into a greased loaf pan. Sprinkle with remaining Parmesan cheese. Bake for 45–55 minutes or until firm and browned on top.

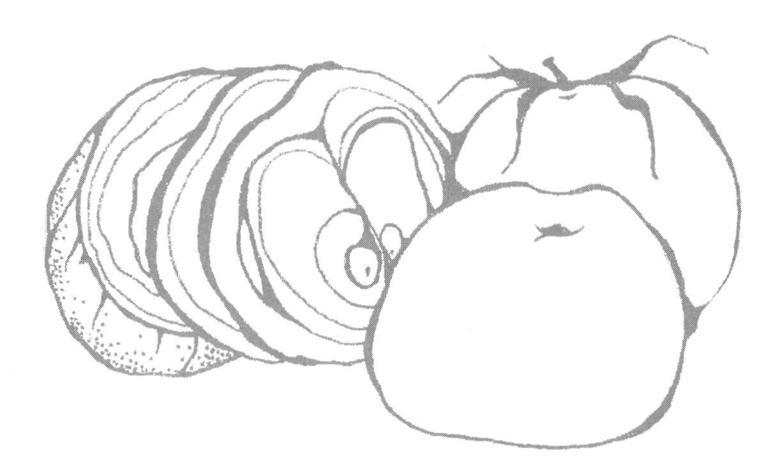

Murg Palak (Indian Chicken with Spinach)

Serves 4

⅓ cup canola oil
1 lb onion, thinly sliced
2 medium tomatoes, cut into wedges
2 bay leaves
4 garlic cloves, minced
1-inch ginger root, grated
1 tablespoon cumin
1 tablespoon coriander
1 tablespoon turmeric
1 tablespoon cayenne
1 ¼ tablespoons salt
½ tablespoon sugar
½ cup plain yogurt
10-oz package frozen spinach, thawed and squeezed dry
4 chicken leg quarters, cut into drumstick and thigh pieces, skinned

Our friend Sikha is a Bengali native who consistently wows us with her food preparations! This dish comes by special request—though all of her dishes are great, if we could only pick one to include as a comfort food, this is it! The combination of aromatic spices wafting from your kitchen will have the neighbors begging for an invitation to dinner!

In a large pot or Dutch oven, heat the oil over medium heat. Add the onion and sauté for 8 minutes, until golden brown. Add the tomatoes and sauté for 5 minutes. Add the bay leaves. Crush the garlic and ginger together with a mortar and pestle and add to the pot. Sauté for 5 minutes. Add the cumin, coriander, turmeric, cayenne, salt, sugar, yogurt, and mix well. Add the spinach and cook, stirring occasionally, for 6–7 minutes. Cut a slit into each of the chicken pieces and add to the pot. Stir until well mixed, cover, and reduce heat to medium-low. Cover and cook until chicken is tender, about 20 minutes. Check the mixture for consistency—it should be like a thick gravy. If it's too moist, uncover and increase the heat for 5 minutes; if it's too dry, add ¼ cup water. Serve over basmati rice.

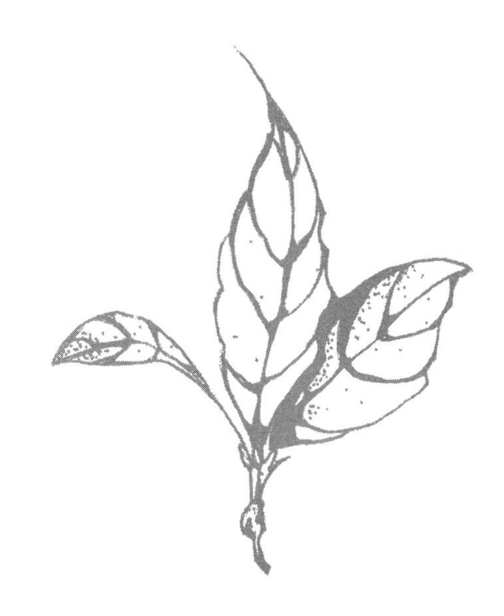

Gambretti Monica (Shrimp Monica)

Serves 2, generously!

This recipe comes from Melissa's brother-in-law, Michael, who has dedicated it to his wife (my sister!) Monica. Michael is a fantastic cook, as one would expect from a graduate of the Culinary Institute of America.

Equipment

3 ½-qt ovenproof sauteuse (Straight sided frying pan) with lid (alternatively, use a casserole pan that you can start on the stove and put into the oven)
cutting board
knife
measuring cup
strainer

Ingredients

1 lb fresh or frozen small shrimp (36–42 or even smaller)
¾ oz (1 bunch) fresh basil
¾ oz (1 bunch) fresh oregano
1 bunch fresh Italian parsley
2 large plum tomatoes
¾ oz dried porcini (cepes) mushrooms
8-oz bottle of clam juice
1 whole head of garlic
1 cup raw rice (Basmati or similar)
extra virgin olive oil
kosher salt
fresh ground black pepper

Preheat the oven to 350°F. Chop the herbs and put aside. Quarter the tomatoes, remove the seeds and pulp, and chop coarsely. Put aside. Thinly slice the garlic and put aside.

Place the mushrooms in a bowl. Add 1 cup of boiling water to the mushrooms and allow to steep.

Add olive oil enough to cover the bottom of the pan to about ⅛-inch deep. Heat the pan and oil a few minutes on medium heat. Add the garlic and sweat until it just turns a little transparent, but do not brown it. Add the shrimp and sauté until just pink, but still undercooked. Add the raw rice and stir, coating each grain of rice in the olive oil.

Allow the rice to heat. While the rice is heating, strain the water from the mushrooms into a measuring cup. Add enough water to bring this to a full cup. Add to the pot. Add the 8 oz of clam juice. Add the tomatoes and mushrooms. Stir and allow to come to a gentle boil. Add the chopped herbs. Add salt and pepper to taste. Cover. Remove from the heat and put into a 350°F oven. Allow to cook, covered and undisturbed, for 22 minutes.

Remove from the oven and check to see that all the liquid is absorbed and the rice is al dente tender. Check it, but do not disturb it any more than needed to check it. If not done, place back in the oven, again covered, for a minute or three. Remove from the oven, fluff and mix with a fork, and serve.

Buono Appetito!

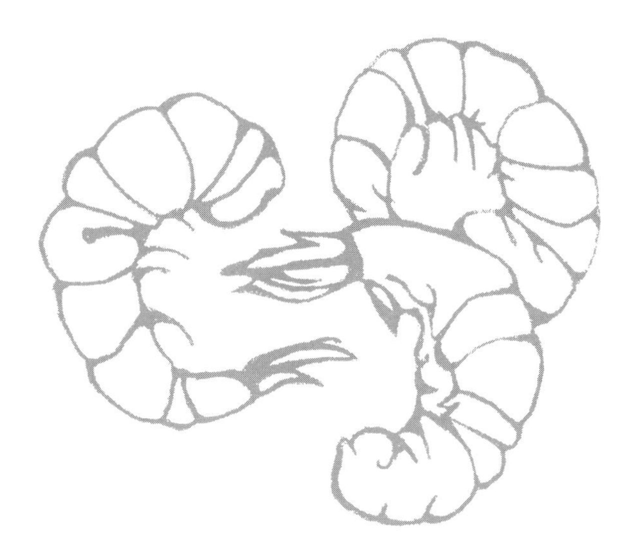

Peggy's Southern Comfort Gumbo

Serves 6–8

Gumbo is a true southern classic abounding with fabulous flavors. This version from our friend Peggy, a native Georgian is sure to be a crowd pleaser.

1 cup oil
¾ cup flour
2 cups chopped onion
1 cup chopped celery
1 cup chopped red bell peppers
6 cloves chopped garlic
¼ tablespoon cayenne
¼ tablespoon ground pepper
1 tablespoon fresh thyme, chopped
1 tablespoon fresh oregano, chopped
2 tablespoons Worcestershire sauce
4 bay leaves
1 lb boneless, skinless chicken thighs, cut into half-inch chunks
1 lb andouille sausage cut into half-inch slices
1 lb chopped kale
1 cup dark beer
1 ½ cups chicken broth
Salt to taste
Tabasco to taste

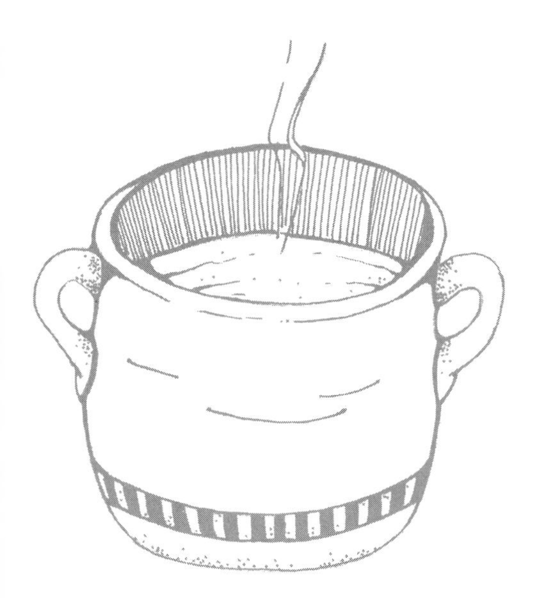

First you start with the roux. This is the key to the gumbo. Combine the oil and the flour in a cast-iron skillet over medium heat. Stir constantly for 20–25 minutes until dark, like chocolate. When this is done, add the onions, celery and peppers and cook about 5 minutes until limp. Add the garlic and chicken and brown for about 5 minutes. Transfer to a large Dutch pan. Add the seasonings and the sausage, kale, beer and broth, stirring to incorporate the liquid into the roux. Lower heat to simmer and add the lemon and salt to taste. Cover and let simmer for 90 minutes, stirring occasionally. Remove bay leaves and lemon. Serve over cooked rice and add Tabasco to taste.

Posole

Serves 6

1 onion, chopped
1 head garlic, whole, unpeeled
2 bay leaves
1 chicken, cut into serving pieces
2 lb pork shoulder meat, cut into serving pieces
1 can hominy (114 oz)
1 can red enchilada sauce (64 oz)

shredded cabbage
radish slices
minced onion
lemon wedges

Posole is a traditional Mexican soup that is warming to both the palate and the soul! This recipe comes to us from our friend Margarita, who needs to be reminded to make it for us more often.

In a large stockpot, place the onion, garlic, bay leaves, chicken, and pork and fill with water to about 5 inches from the top. Bring to a boil, then reduce heat to medium and cook until the meat is cooked, about 30 minutes. Drain the hominy and add to the pot. When the hominy is tender, add the enchilada sauce and salt to taste and simmer for 5–10 minutes. Carefully remove the head of garlic. Ladle the soup into large bowls and garnish with shredded cabbage, radish slices, minced onion and a wedge of lemon. Serve with warm corn tortillas.

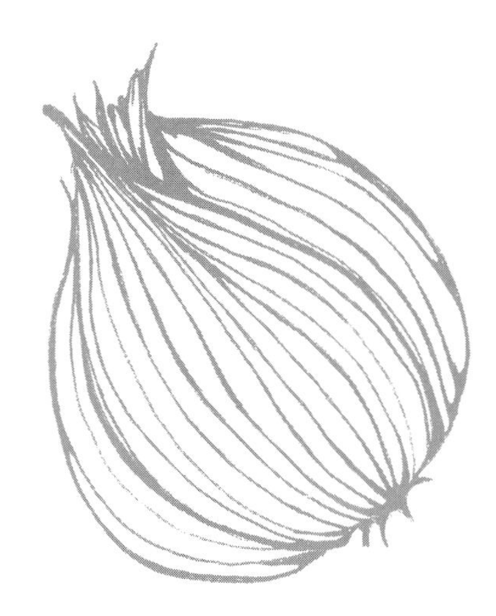

Shepherd's Pie

Serves 6

This is such a quintessential comfort food that we wonder why we don't see it more often! The inspiration for this version comes from our friends Robert and Syd who remind us that some foods are designated as "comfort" for a reason.

2 tablespoons olive oil
1 onion, chopped
1 cup sliced mushrooms
1 ¼ lb ground turkey
1 cup frozen peas
1 cup frozen corn
1 tablespoon minced sage
1 tablespoon minced rosemary
½ cup chicken broth
¼ cup dry white wine
1 tablespoon flour
2 tablespoons water
2 cups shredded cheddar cheese
2 lb mashed potatoes

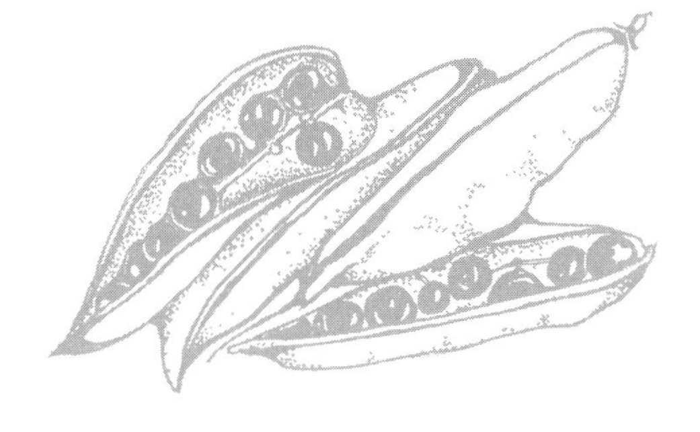

Preheat oven to 375°F. In a large skillet, heat the oil over medium heat. Sauté the onions for 3 minutes, add the mushrooms and cook for an additional 3 minutes. Add the ground turkey and cook, breaking up the meat, until it is no longer pink. Stir in the vegetables, herbs, broth, and wine and bring to a simmer. In a small bowl, make a slurry of the flour and water, and stir into the meat mixture. Bring back to a simmer, and then remove from heat. Transfer the meat mixture to a baking dish (an oval gratin dish works well). Spread the cheese evenly over the top of the filling. Cover the cheese with the mashed potatoes—an easy way to do this is to spoon the potatoes into a plastic Ziploc bag, cut out one of the corners of the bag, and pipe the potatoes over the dish. Smooth the potatoes with the back of a spoon to cover the top of the dish completely. Bake for 45 minutes. If you want a darker crust on the potatoes, put the dish under a broiler for a couple of minutes, but be sure to keep an eye on it so it doesn't burn!

Soupe au Pistou

Serves 4

¾ cup fresh basil leaves
3 tablespoons pine nuts
⅓ cup olive oil

1 leek, diced
2 carrots, diced
1 potato, diced
2 tablespoons fresh thyme
6 cups vegetable broth
1 zucchini, diced
1 tomato, diced
2 cups white kidney beans (canned, drained)
shaved parmesan

Emmanuelle remembers:

"My grandmother used to make this soup for us when we visited her in Cannes every summer. It is an instant pleasure to the olfactory senses! If you want the ultimate experience, grind the pistou with a mortar and pestle instead of using a food processor. My grandmother would give us each a turn grinding the mixture so that the result was truly a family effort!"

For the Pistou

In a food processor, pulse together the fresh basil and the pine nuts until coarsely chopped. With the motor running, stream in the olive oil and process until smooth.

For the Soup

In a large stockpot, combine the leek, carrot, potato, and thyme. Cover with the vegetable broth, bring to a simmer and cook for 15 minutes. Add the zucchini, tomato, and beans, and cook for an additional 5 minutes.

Immediately before serving, add the pistou to the soup and stir. Serve the soup in large bowls, garnished with the shaved parmesan.

Sage and Potato Gratin

Serves 6

We've never met a gratin that we didn't like—and this is no exception! The aromas that waft from the oven as it cooks envelop you in a sense of warmth and peace. Incidentally, it tastes great, too!

2 tablespoons olive oil
4 lb potatoes, peeled and sliced
1 ½ cups heavy cream
1 cup milk
1 lb smoked mozzarella, grated
¼ cup chopped sage
1 cup grated parmesan
salt and pepper

Preheat oven to 375°F. Coat the bottom and sides of a 9 x 13 glass baking dish with the oil. In a large bowl, toss the potato slices with salt and pepper. Combine the cream and milk in a measuring cup. Place a layer of potato slices into the dish. Top with ⅓ of the mozzarella, ⅓ of the sage, and ⅓ of the cream mixture. Continue layering, finishing with a top layer of potatoes. Cover the top of the potatoes with the parmesan. Bake for 60–90 minutes, until the potatoes are very soft. Let sit for 10 minutes before serving.

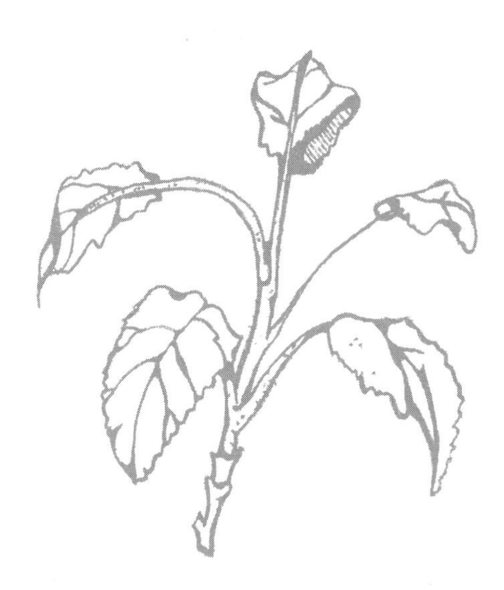

Herbed Spaghetti Squash Casserole

Serves 4

1 spaghetti squash
¾ cup chopped onion
2 garlic cloves, crushed or minced
2 chopped tomatoes
1 cup mushrooms, sliced
½ tablespoon thyme
½ tablespoon oregano
½ tablespoon savory
1 tablespoon basil
1 cup ricotta cheese
¾ cup breadcrumbs
1 cup parmesan cheese
1 cup grated Swiss cheese

The combination of the thyme, oregano, savory and basil cooking in the oven will forever remind me of cold evenings when my (Emmanuelle's) mother would make this for our family. It is hearty, but not heavy. It will surely become one of your family's favorites, too!

Preheat oven to 400°F. Cut squash in half and remove seeds. Place cut side down onto an oiled baking sheet and bake for 30 minutes. Remove from oven and cool until able to handle. Reduce oven heat to 350°F. Using a fork, scrape the flesh of the squash into spaghetti-like strands into a large bowl. Sauté onion, tomato, garlic, mushrooms and herbs for 10 minutes. Add to squash along with the ricotta, parmesan and breadcrumbs. Mix well and turn into a lightly oiled casserole dish. Top with Swiss cheese and bake for 50 minutes.

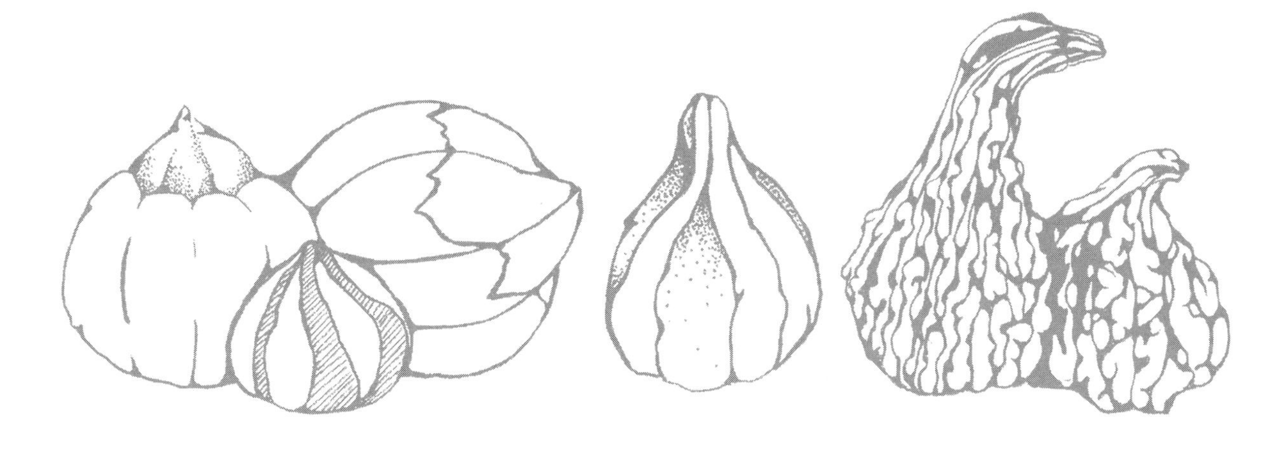

Mum's Cornbread Dressing

Serves 6

This classic southern dish comes to us from our friend Peggy, a great cook who has been nice enough to share several of her favorite southern recipes for comfort foods.

"This is the recipe from my mother's mother and has been served at every Thanksgiving and Christmas we have had in our family. It is tradition in the south that you don't stuff the turkey but cook the dressing outside the bird, hence it is called dressing not stuffing. You need a cast iron skillet for this to get the brown crust that makes this dressing special."

Dressing

1 pan of cornbread (recipe follows)
1 large onion, chopped
3 celery stalks, chopped
4 garlic cloves, minced
4 biscuits or 5 slices of bread
water
salt & pepper to taste
2 tablespoons turmeric
2 tablespoons minced fresh sage
1 tablespoon minced fresh thyme
1 tablespoon minced oregano
1 egg
1 tablespoon baking powder
vegetable oil

Take a large bowl and break up the cornbread and biscuits/bread into it. Put in onion, celery, garlic, sage, turmeric, thyme, oregano and salt and pepper to taste. Put in enough water to reach about halfway and then mix everything together. Cover and let sit overnight. The next day, stir again and check for consistency. It should be moist but not overly runny. Add more water if needed. Right before you are going to cook the dressing, add the egg and baking powder and stir. Heat a cast iron skillet in the oven at 350°F with 2–3 tablespoons of oil in it. You should heat it about 10–15 minutes until oil is hot. Remove from oven and carefully pour in batter. It might splatter a bit so be careful. The dressing should come up to near the top. Return to oven and bake at 350°F for 45–60 minutes or until browned on the bottom and firm.
Cut into squares and serve. Makes 10–12 servings.

Buttermilk Cornbread

1 cup all purpose flour
1 cup white ground cornmeal
4 tablespoons baking powder
½ teaspoon baking soda
2 tablespoons salt
1 egg
1 ½ cups buttermilk
vegetable oil

Mix all ingredients together. Heat oven to 350°F. Put cornbread into greased cast iron skillet. Bake for 20–25 minutes.

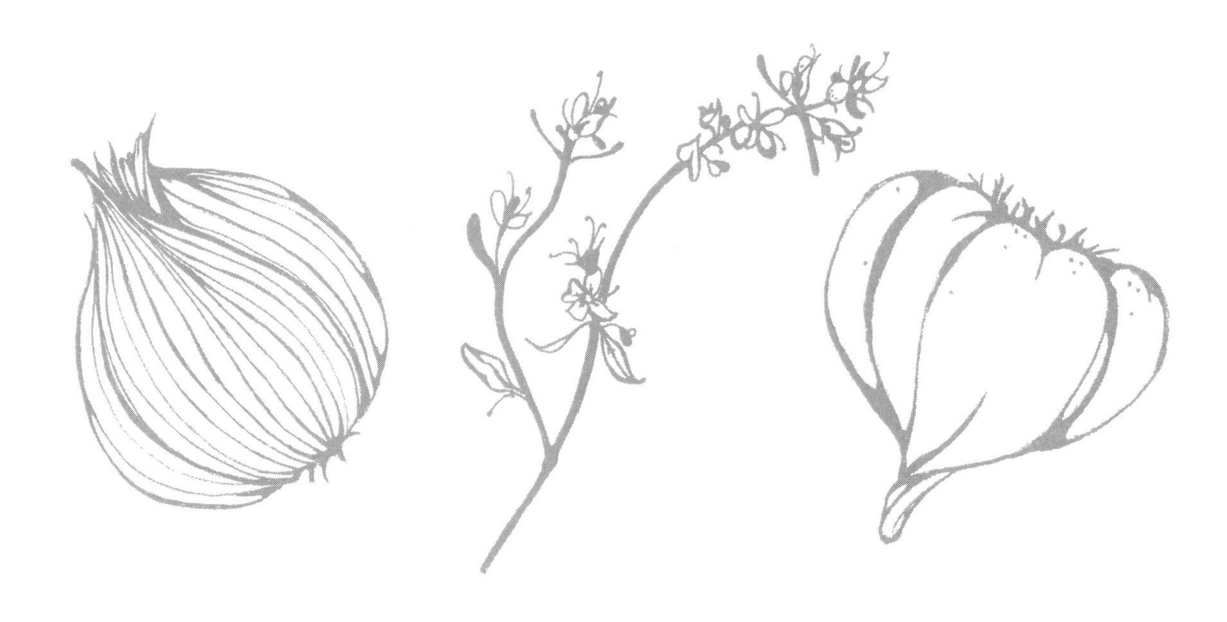

Mikey's Pizza Bianco a la Vongole

This fabulous pizza creation comes from Melissa's brother-in-law Michael, aka Michele, aka Mikey. If you ever wanted pizza instructions from a true Italian chef, look no further! Thanks, Mikey!

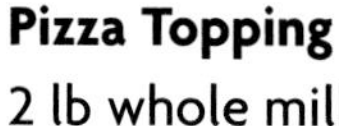

Pizza Topping

2 lb whole milk ricotta cheese
1 lb fresh mozzarella cheese
2 oz grated reggiano romano cheese
2 cans (6–8 ounces each) coarsely chopped clams
1 cup fresh basil leaves
2 cups fresh Italian parsley leaves
1/4 cup fresh oregano leaves
1 whole clove garlic
1 lb frozen chopped spinach
kosher salt
freshly ground black pepper

Ingredient Notes

• Try to find canned clams that have large pieces of meat. You're looking for clams that would be suitable for use in chowder.
• Drain the ricotta for a time if it has water in it. You want the ricotta to be very dry.
• The fresh mozzarella is sold in liquid (whey). It is increasingly available, so you should be able to find it. As a last resort you can use bagged shredded mozzarella, but it isn't really the same product.
• If you choose, you can substitute dried herbs for the fresh herbs. Reduce the amounts accordingly and allow the final mixture to stand for a fair amount of time—even overnight—to allow the dried herbs to rehydrate.

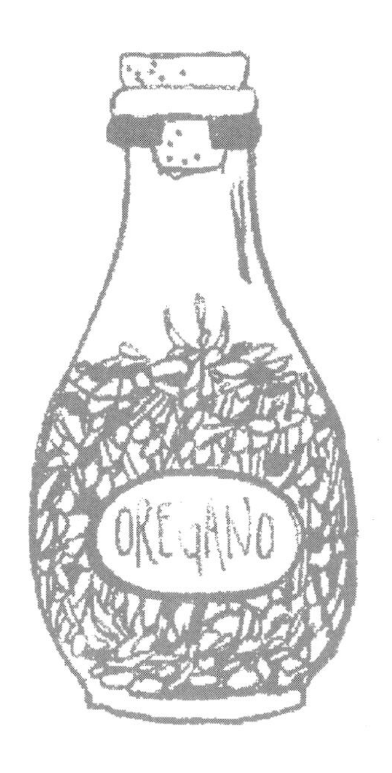

Thaw the spinach. Place the spinach in a sieve or cheesecloth and thoroughly squeeze out all the residual water. When the spinach is very dry, put it in the refrigerator and hold.

Peel and chop the garlic. Put aside. Coarsely chop the herbs. Put aside.

Drain the ricotta and place it into a large mixing bowl. Shred the mozzarella into the bowl with the ricotta. Shred it on the largest-hole side of a cheese grater. The technique is really as much pushing it through the holes as it is grating it. Add the reggiano, garlic, and herbs to the cheese. Drain the clams and squeeze out any remaining liquid. Add to the cheese.

Fold the cheese mixture gently to combine all ingredients. Salt and pepper to taste. Set aside and allow the flavors to blend for a few hours in the refrigerator.

Pizza Dough

3 cups bread flour
½ teaspoon kosher salt
2 tablespoons extra virgin olive oil
2 packages dry yeast
1 cup water at 118°F
1 pinch of sugar

Add the yeast to the water, mix and dissolve with a fork. Add a pinch of sugar to activate the yeast. Set aside for five minutes or until the yeast foams.

Place the flour in the bowl of a mixer with a dough hook. Add the salt and the olive oil. Add the water and yeast mixture. Using the fork used to dissolve the yeast, mix the ingredients to roughly combine them.

Mix the dough with a dough hook on low speed for 10 minutes. Scrape the bowl only if needed. The dough should pull away from the bowl on its own.

Place the dough in a bowl that has been oiled with some olive oil. Turn the dough in the bowl to cover it all around with the oil. Cover the bowl with a towel and allow the dough to proof until double in size (about 45 minutes). Punch the dough down and allow to proof a second time (about 30 minutes).

Assembly and Baking

pizza dough (from above)
pizza topping (from above)
spinach (from above)
bread flour
olive oil
cornmeal

Place a pizza stone in your oven and preheat to 500°F or hotter. Commercial pizza ovens often produce temperatures in excess of 750°F, so make your oven as hot as it can get. Be sure to preheat the oven for a sufficiently long time to ensure that not only the oven, but also the stone, are at maximum temperature. A one hour preheating time is not excessive.

Punch the dough down. Roll it into a roughly cylindrical or loaf shape. Divide the dough into six even portions.

Divide (or imagine dividing) the topping and the spinach into six equal portions, one portion for each of the six dough portions.

Generously flour a cutting board and roll the dough out into a circle. Roll until the dough is quite thin—approximately 1/8 inch thick.

Sprinkle some cornmeal on a wooden pizza peel and transfer the dough to the peel.

Drizzle olive oil on the dough and wipe or brush so as to coat the top of the dough completely, except for a margin at the edge of approximately 1/2 inch, which is left uncoated. Once the olive oil is drizzled on the dough, a pastry brush is very hand for spreading it.

This step is critical in all pizza making, as it prevents the toppings from soaking the dough and making it soggy.

Sprinkle spinach evenly on the dough in small, nut-sized bits.

Drop the topping on the dough, also in small dollops evenly over the entire pizza. It is not necessary to evenly spread the topping. It will flow as it bakes. Just keep the dollops in a more or less even pattern over the surface of the dough. Slide the prepared pizza onto the stone in the oven.

Allow the pizza to bake until the crust is evenly brown (to quite dark brown) at the edges. The pizza will cook in 2–4 minutes, depending on the temperature of your oven and the density of your stone. Remove the pizza from the oven with the peel and allow it to stand for a minute or so before cutting. Cut with a sturdy pizza wheel.

Buono Appetito!

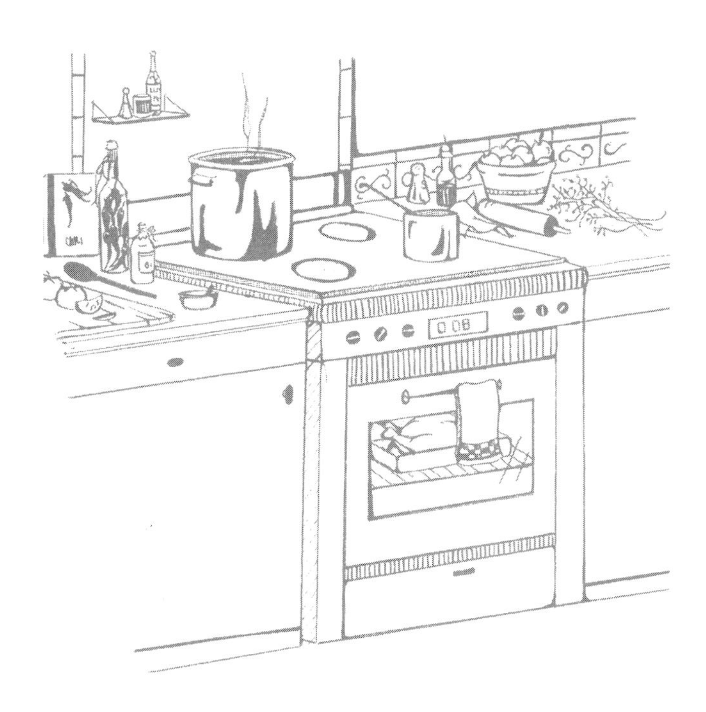

North Woods Rice

Serves 4

This wonderful aromatic dish comes to us from our friend Rob, who manages to take a simple grain such as rice and turn it into a sumptuous dish time and time again, and each time with a different flair. In this version, wild rice, mushrooms, walnuts and sage combine to create a fabulously earthy and soul-soothing creation.

¼ cup canola oil
1 cup chopped onions
½ oz dried wild mushrooms, chopped
½ cup crimini mushrooms, chopped
½ cup chopped walnuts
½ cup wild rice
1 ½ cups long grain rice (jasmine rice, preferred)
½ tablespoon sage, minced
5 cups water
1 tablespoon Worcestershire sauce
1 carrot, cut into strips
1 cup petit peas, fresh or frozen, thawed
salt and pepper to taste

In a 2-quart saucepan, heat the oil over medium-high heat. Sauté the onions until they just become translucent. Add the mushrooms, walnuts, wild rice, white rice and sage, and stir until well coated with the oil. Cook until the rice just starts to turn golden, stirring. Add the water and Worcestershire, cover and bring to a boil. Reduce heat to a simmer, add the carrots, cover and cook until the liquid is almost all absorbed. Stir in the peas, season with salt and pepper, and return to low, covered, until all of the liquid is absorbed. Remove from heat and let sit for 5 minutes. Stir and serve!

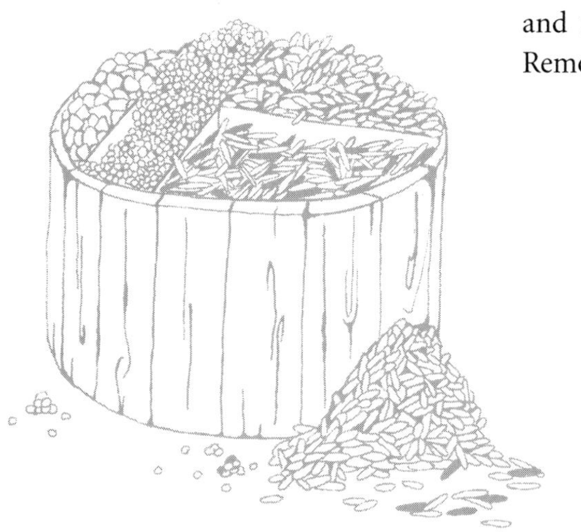

Vanilla Bean Bread Pudding with Meringue

1 qt whole milk
1 whole vanilla bean
1 loaf stale French bread
3 eggs
2 cups sugar
2 tablespoons melted margarine

3 egg whites
3 tablespoons sugar

This is a favorite of our good friend Tonya, who writes:

"Whenever my sister or I were sick when we were little girls, our mother made us treats. You could always count on soft-boiled eggs followed by tapioca pudding, rice pudding, or bread pudding. As the years went by and we learned to cook, we began experimenting with our mother's recipe for bread pudding. After eating more bread pudding than we care to admit, we finally came up with the most fragrant vanilla bread pudding ever!"

Pour milk into a 2-quart saucepan. Split vanilla bean lengthwise, and add to the milk. Simmer on low heat for 20 minutes—do not boil! Remove from heat and cool, refrigerated, for one hour.

Preheat oven to 350°F. While the milk cools, tear the bread into 1-inch pieces and place into a 3-quart baking dish. Remove the vanilla bean from the cooled milk. In a small bowl, whisk the eggs together with the sugar and melted margarine. Whisk the egg mixture into the milk, and pour over the bread. Place the pan in the oven and bake for 55 minutes.

Just before the pudding is finished baking, prepare the meringue. Place the egg whites in a chilled, clean metal bowl, and whisk until soft peaks are formed. Add the sugar, and continue whisking until the peaks are stiff.

Remove the pudding from the oven, and increase the oven temperature to 450°F. Spread the meringue evenly over the bread pudding. Bake for an additional 5 minutes, or until the meringue is browned.

Orange and Apricot Clafouti with Crème Anglaise

Clafouti is a classic French dessert. This is a version of Emmanuelle's grandmother's recipe, replacing the traditional whole cherries with fresh apricots.

Clafouti

2 tablespoons butter
4 eggs
⅓ cup orange blossom honey
1 vanilla bean, split lengthwise
2 tablespoons butter, melted
1 tablespoon Grand Marnier
1 cup flour
1 ½ cups milk
1 ½ lbs fresh apricots, quartered
½ cup sugar

Preheat oven to 350°F. In a mixing bowl, whisk the eggs and honey. Scrape the vanilla bean into the egg mixture. Stir in the butter and Grand Marnier. Whisk in the milk until smooth. In a separate bowl, toss the apricots with the sugar. Place the apricots in a baking dish. Pour the batter over the apricots and bake for 40–45 minutes, or until a knife inserted into the cake comes out clean. Remove from oven and cool for 5 minutes. Serve with crème Anglaise (recipe follows).

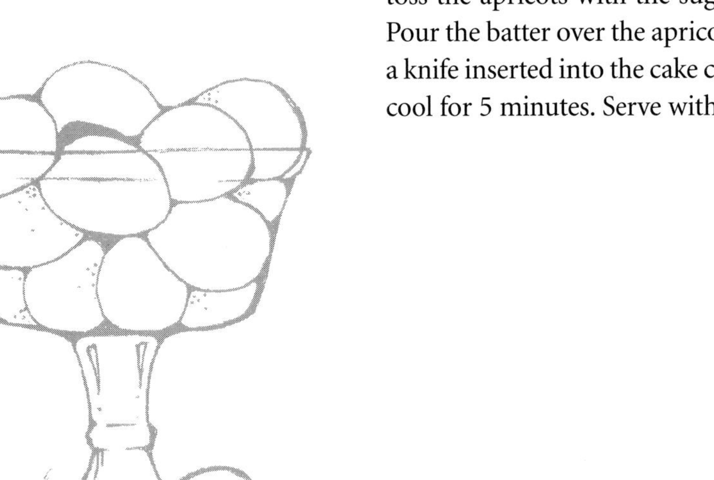

Crème Anglaise
3 cups milk
1 cup heavy cream
2 vanilla beans, split lengthwise
12 egg yolks
½ cup sugar

In a saucepan, combine the milk, cream, and vanilla beans. Bring to a simmer over medium heat. In a mixing bowl, whisk the egg yolks with the sugar. Slowly whisk one cup of the heated milk to the egg mixture. Whisk the eggs back into the rest of the hot milk, reduce heat to low, and stir until the custard coats the back of a spoon. Remove vanilla beans and scrape the paste from the pods into the custard. Cool slightly before serving.

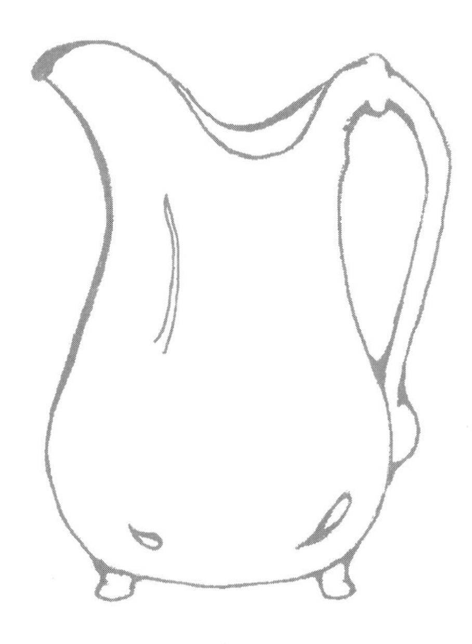

Chai Tea

This comes to us from our friend Teresa, a self-professed ex-hippie from San Francisco!

"Chai is a strong, sweet, spiced tea from India that is gaining popularity in the United States. You can now find tea bags which say "chai" but it is well worth the effort to make it from scratch. My sister taught me how to make chai after she returned from spending nine months in India. If your family is home when you make this, you may want to double the recipe as the aroma of the cooking spices will bring them into the kitchen to inquire what you are making! My 14-year-old son recently acclaimed that this is 'the best drink ever'."

3 cups water
4 Earl Grey tea bags
⅛-inch slice of fresh ginger
8 whole dried cardamom pods
3 whole cloves
1 cinnamon stick, split lengthwise
¼ cup half and half
¼ cup milk
3 tablespoons sugar

Bring water to a boil in a saucepan. Reduce the heat to low, and add the tea bags and spices. Stir well, then cover. The tea should be at a low simmer, but not boiling. Let cook for 3 minutes. Use a spoon to press the cardamom pods against the sides of the saucepan to break them open. Cook for 2 minutes. Using a strainer, scoop the tea bags and spices out of the tea. Add the half and half, milk, and sugar. Cook for 2 more minutes, stirring occasionally, until the tea is hot. Serve immediately.

Resource Guide

Here are some of our recommendations for books, magazine and Internet sites to help you further explore the worlds of aromatherapy and cooking!

Publications on Aromatherapy and Herbs

Aromatherapy and the Mind: Julia Lawless
Aromatherapy for Dummies: Kathy Keville
The Aromatherapy Book: Jeanne Rose
The Complete Book of Essential Oils & Aromatherapy: Valerie Ann Worwood
Aromatherapy; The Complete Guide to Plant and Flower Essences for Health and Beauty: Daniele Ryman
Rodale's Illustrated Encyclopedia of Herbs: Kowalchik & Hylton, Eds.
Aromatherapy Magazine (www.aromatherapymagazine.com)

Internet Sites for Aromatherapy

If you search out any other sites, be sure to check that the oils they supply are organic!

www.herbproducts.com
www.penzeys.com
www.essentialoils.com
www.apothecary-shoppe.com
www.naha.org (National Association for Holistic Aromatherapy)
www.aromaweb.com

Internet Sites for Kitchen Equipment

www.restaurant-store.com
www.chefscatalog.com
www.surlatable.com
www.crateandbarrel.com
www.williamssonoma.com

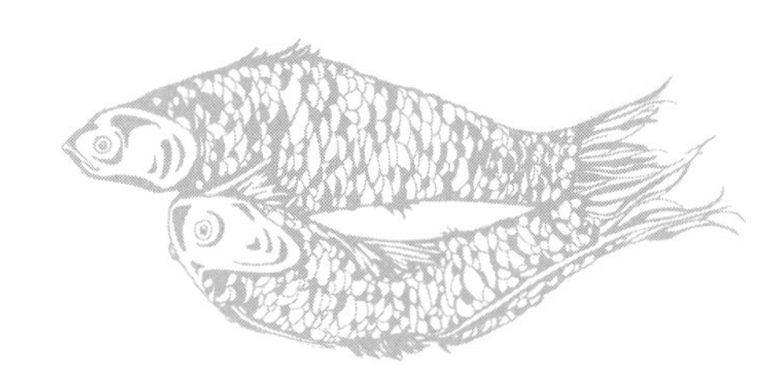

Index

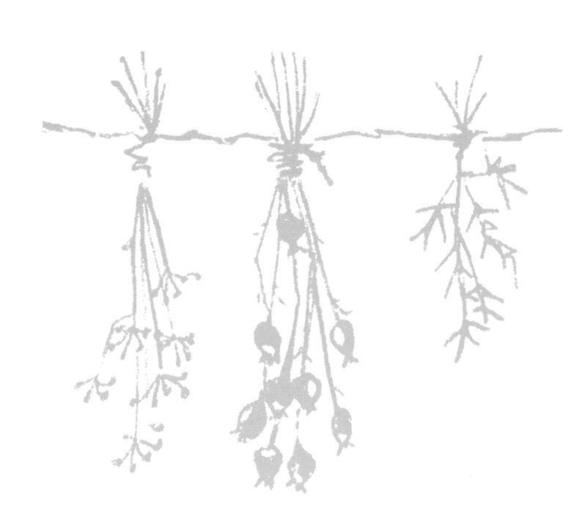

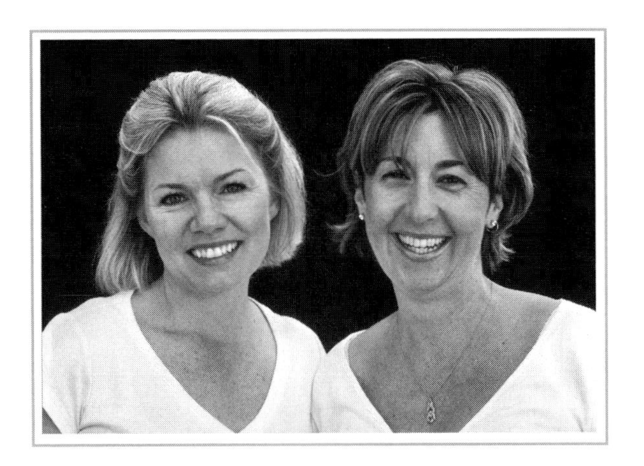

About the Authors

Lifelong food fanatics **Melissa Dale** and **Emmanuelle Lipsky** have been sharing a passion for life, friendship, and all things culinary for over twenty years. They are essentially "home cooks," but have built upon their culinary foundations through numerous cooking courses, including the Pro Chef I program at the Epicurean School of Culinary Arts in Los Angeles. They have also become increasingly interested in the practice of aromatherapy, incorporating the therapeutic benefits of plant essences into their daily lives. The fusion of these two interests was the impetus for this book.

The authors' cooking philosophy is fairly simple and hardly unique: use the freshest ingredients available, keep the preparation straightforward, and don't be afraid to experiment with new things! Although their cooking is quite healthful, they don't exactly shy away from the occasional use of butter, cream, and wine in their cooking. Remember that age-old motto of moderation in all things! Melissa and Emmanuelle also believe that a little bit of self-indulgence is a good thing, so don't be afraid to enjoy a little cream sauce now and then. Their advice? Just do a couple of extra sit-ups, and you'll be fine . . .

As for the authors' personal backgrounds, Melissa is a native New Englander whose day job as a water quality chemist includes participating on a flavor profile panel. Tasting water is not as much fun as tasting food, but it does help to keep the taste buds alert! Emmanuelle was born and raised in Paris, and came to the U.S. for college, which is where she and Melissa met. Emmanuelle earned her masters degree in psychology, which comes in handy in her position as a junior high school teacher! Currently, Melissa and Emmanuelle both reside in southern California.